So
Your
Doctor
Recommended
Surgery

So Your Doctor Recommended Surgery

JOHN LEWIS, M.D.

An Owl Book
Henry Holt and Company   New York

Library of Congress Cataloging-in-Publication Data
Lewis, John, M.D.
So your doctor recommended surgery / John Lewis. —
1st Owl book ed.
p.   cm.
"An Owl book."
Reprint. Originally published: New York: Dembner Books, © 1990.
Includes bibliographical references and index.
1. Surgery—Popular works.   2. Surgery—Decision making.
3. Surgery, Unnecessary—Popular works.   4. Patient education.
I. Title.
RD31.3.L49   1991
617—dc20   91-22090
                                                                            CIP
ISBN 0-8050-1683-X (An Owl Book: pbk.)

Henry Holt books are available at special discounts
for bulk purchases for sales promotions, premiums,
fund-raising, or educational use. Special editions
or book excerpts can also be created to specification.
For details contact:
Special Sales Director, Henry Holt and Company, Inc.,
115 West 18th Street, New York, New York 10011.

First published in hardcover by Red Dembner Enterprises Corp.
in 1990.

First Owl Book Edition—1992

Printed in the United States of America
Recognizing the importance of preserving the written word,
Henry Holt and Company, Inc., by policy, prints all of its
first editions on acid-free paper. ∞

1   3   5   7   9   10   8   6   4   2

It is your body. It is your life. The final decision is yours

George Crile, Jr., M.D.

Contents

Preface

Agitated by what they refer to as an economic crisis in medical care, those who pay the bill have discovered a lot of unnecessary medical intervention and treatment. In particular, they find surgery often not needed. We've known this for a long time, of course, but now in order to reduce the waste, various agencies—government, private insurers, and employers—have come up with plans that demand response from a previously sluggish profession. My profession, which finds itself at the onset of a revolution—its social, political, economic, ethical, and scientific character being wrenched into new forms.

If this revolution achieves a rational and waste-free system, designed clearly in your favor, you may some day be able to enter it in simple trust. Not yet, however—perhaps never. An explicit recognition that you, the patient, are expected to question, to accept responsibility, to take charge, has become part of the medical process. Informed consent, despite some erudite objections, has become an ethical principle for the profession. Doctors practice it, so must you. You will survive best in the system if you acquire pertinent information before you consent to surgery.

This book provides specific information in separate chapters about the most frequent, elective surgical operations. Of more general interest are the first two chapters and the last four. You might consider reading the first two, then the chapter concerned with the operation your doctor has recommended; follow this with any or all of the last chapters.

Three main entities and their interactions are considered throughout the book: patients, doctors, and surgical operations. My comments on them are based upon my experience as a surgeon, my exposure as a patient, and my reading.

Patients, I believe, often have an unjustified trust in surgery. They accept a dangerous personal invasion with surprising ignorance of surgeons and the nature of surgery.

Doctors, it seems to me, work with a (sometimes unrecognized) lack of sound data, though they usually intend well. In the ways they publicly advocate their services, they attribute too much value to doctor visits, hospital care, and intervention. Furthermore, their profession suffers a critical gap between its medical scientists and its practitioners. (Fortunately, this may become smaller as the revolution I mentioned encourages the scientific impulse.)

Surgical operations, though often technically brilliant, are too frequently unsupported by clear evidence that they are needed.

Your natural expectation that these entities will blend smoothly together—in particular that surgery's two main actors, doctor and patient, have parallel objectives—may fail. These and other matters discussed in the book should encourage you to shoulder more responsibility—perhaps more than you might have wanted. But the better you are informed, the less you will risk. This book intends to help you in that task—and also, perhaps, to interest you in surgery's odd and lively venture.

The medical literature has been an important source for the text, providing many analyses of surgical folly and success. The profession, you see, is not entirely a monolith in defense of old dogma; rebels are common and vocal.

When I have referred to specific medical or nonmedical sources, I have done so with the author-date system. Within the text the author's last name and the date of publication are given in parentheses (Smith, 1988). This is keyed to "References" at the end of the book, an alphabetically arranged list of all the works cited.

The case histories scattered through the book, although based on real experiences, have been superficially fictionalized, in order to avoid invasion of privacy.

Medical jargon is unavoidable in a book like this. I have attempted to clarify terms with brief parenthetical definitions at first encounter.

Acknowledgments

I'm grateful to the many teachers, colleagues, students, patients, and friends who, in various ways over the years, molded the frame of mind that has led to this book, but I won't try to list them. Here I want to acknowledge the help of a few individuals who contributed more directly and recently to the project: Max Gartenberg who set me on the right course; Fred Preston, George Higgins, and Art Rink who guided or refreshed my medical understanding; Evelyn Fay and her library associates who provided most of the published sources; Winifred Brode, Barbara Withey, Charles Newman, Beulah Englesberg, and Marina Alzugaray who furnished editorial help or special information; and my wife, Ruth, for a long career of gracious support.

The points of view and opinions in the book are mine. Don't blame those whose help I have acknowledged; they are not responsible. I do believe, however, that many thoughtful individuals, including many surgeons, hold a questioning, skeptical opinion of surgery similar to the one that permeates this book.

1

So Your Doctor Recommended Surgery

A doctor's intentions are usually good. Your doctor probably believes he is acting in your best interest when he recommends surgery, but there are times—unfortunately too many—when this proves not to be so.

Take the case of J.N., an internist friend of mine. Three months after his sixty-fifth birthday he was experiencing nagging chest pain and general lassitude. When he complained to his partner and said he thought he'd go home early, the partner took an electrocardiograph and found definite signs of a heart attack.

J.N. stopped work for a couple of weeks, and then slowly returned to a full schedule. He felt pretty good, took some medicines, and had no angina, but the problem preyed on his mind. He went to a cardiologist at a large midwestern clinic where X rays of his coronary arteries showed a narrowing that could, technically, be bypassed surgically. The operation wasn't really necessary, said the cardiologist, because there was no evidence that he'd live longer or avoid future attacks by having it.

But a cardiac surgeon was a little more encouraging; the heart would probably pump better afterward if J.N. had the operation, he said. J.N. decided to have the surgery. He probably believed that the quality of his life would thereby be enhanced. Postoperatively his blood pressure fell, and he failed to regain consciousness. For three months he existed in a comatose or semicomatose state. Slowly he recovered. He hasn't been able to resume his practice, but he reads, plans to write his memoirs, and exercises a little every day.

Surgeons have always performed unnecessary surgery, surely not intentionally, but nonetheless industriously. When they have a hard time deciding what treatment, if any, is best, doctors may recommend surgery. And it seems that our species has an enormous appetite for it. Until recently we allowed a million tonsillectomies a year—almost all useless—to be performed on our children.

Of course you may really need the operation your doctor has recommended. Surgeons have devised many excellent, lifesaving or life-improving operations. Which ones are the good ones? How can you avoid useless operations, escape unnecessary risk? How can you tell if the operation recommended for you suits your condition? This book intends to help you answer these questions. You may jump directly to the chapter on a particular surgical operation or, better still, read on.

WHY SURGERY?

As a definitive solution, surgery may seem the best course. "When in doubt take it out," the confident surgeon tells himself, his colleagues, and his patients. Stop the pills, forget the tiresome hygiene, and go under the knife—at only a small, but never zero, risk. Why not? you think. Maybe a friend of yours had your identical complaint—miserable, unrelenting—and now he . . . Can you believe it? Bud is back playing tennis. You remember how it was? He could hardly hobble around the court. Arthritis. He had his hip joint replaced. Nothing to it.

CAUTION, PLEASE

So, surgery sounds like a reasonable, even an exciting, option. But note: a few years ago a House Subcommittee on Oversight and Investigation determined that there were some 10,000 deaths a year in this country due to unnecessary surgery (Subcommittee on Oversight, 1978). That's probably an underestimation. Don't be enticed into accepting a useless and possibly dangerous operation by your surgeon's enthusiasm for his craft and your own optimistic expectations. You may be fooled. You could be killed.

Often we expect too much of surgery, and end up with a scar more painful than the disability for which we had the operation. Our body's relentless way of aging or, regrettably, our irreversible disability may prevent complete surgical restoration. Or the malady for which we seek a cure may not yet, despite modern medicine's spectacular discoveries, have a first-class treatment. Many surgical operations represent what Lewis Thomas, medical scientist, former president of the Sloan-Kettering Center, and prize-winning author of *Lives of a Cell* (1971), has called a "halfway technology."

He described three technological levels in medicine. The first is the care that tides patients through diseases that are not well understood and have no specific treatments. Sometimes called "supportive therapy," care at this level is important, expensive, and time-consuming. The second level, "halfway technology," represents the kind of therapies that must be done to compensate for diseases whose course medicine is unable to do very much about. Artificial organ implantations are dazzling surgical examples; many operations that are the result of impressive technical achievement are at this level of technology. The third level of technology, though less noticeable, is the genuinely decisive technology, the real high technology of modern medicine. Immunizations against diphtheria and childhood virus diseases and the use of antibiotics for bacterial infections are examples.

Some years ago L.N., a thirty-three-year-old farmer who had lain in a Veteran's hospital bed for six months, was told that his tuberculosis was now stable—but, of course, not cured. L.N.'s sputum was still positive for the tubercle bacillus, and X rays showed a cavity in the right upper lung. His case had been presented at the weekly conference of local authorities, and it was recommended that he have the diseased part of his lung removed after suitable preparation with the newly discovered antibiotic, streptomycin. L.N. agreed to the recommendation. His immediate postoperative recovery was satisfactory, but a week after surgery he ran a fever. The surgeons identified an infection within the chest at the operative site (an empyema) and implanted a tube to drain it. Later several ribs had to be taken out in order to close the cavity left by the infection.

Just at the time when L.N. was finally ready to leave the hospital, six months after surgery, with his tuberculosis satisfactorily arrested, several publications appeared in the medical literature showing that antibiotics alone were adequate treatment for cases such as his. L.N. had undergone an operation that represented halfway technology. It seemed the best that could be done at the time, but it was replaced by a simpler, less radical, less expensive, and more effective treatment—the decisive or high technology Thomas referred to. Had L.N. and his doctors waited a little longer he would certainly have been better off.

Surgery for cancer, coronary bypass, and such sensational surgical efforts as major-organ transplantations are present-day examples of halfway technology: Often complex and difficult, the best that medicine can provide now, they are by no means ideal. We can expect that halfway technologies will be replaced when medical science learns more about how to prevent, immunize against, or otherwise treat the disease. Less expensive, less risky, and more effective procedures than surgery will win out.

QUALITY

Despite the good intentions of surgeons and almost everyone else connected with the surgical enterprise, surgery lacks adequate quality control. Neither the medical profession nor the government nor the hospital has yet provided it. The Joint Commission on Accreditation of Hospitals, for example, checks on the organizational structure of a hospital and the way it carries out its functions before they will approve it, but it doesn't check on the final and most critical issue to you, the results. The commission makes sure that the hospital has surgical conferences and complete medical records—all to the good—but it ignores the complication rates and the mortality rates—statistics it has apparently found too touchy. Only recently has it shown an interest in developing ways of measuring "outcomes."

If the hospital system doesn't guarantee surgical quality control, you might imagine that control would have fallen under some organized national system, in the way that drugs have fallen under the Food and Drug Administration (FDA). It hasn't. Before accepting a drug for general use, the FDA requires "substantial evidence consisting of adequate and well-controlled investigations," including "a method of selection" that "assigns subjects to test groups in such a way as to minimize bias."

Trials designed to provide that kind of evidence have improved clinical medicine. Many of us will remember how the FDA saved us from thalidomide and an epidemic of birth defects in the 1960s. Critics have complained that the FDA had denied us some important drugs (such as propranolol and new drugs for AIDS) longer than necessary, but altogether its record is excellent. Before lovastatin, a promising new drug to lower blood cholesterol and thus the risk of heart attacks, was released for general use, tests had to convince the FDA of its effectiveness and safety. Surgery lacks this kind of control. The coronary bypass operation was used in this country for several years (from 1967 to 1972) before investigators started the first controlled clinical test. And use of the operation has never been regulated, except voluntarily, by the results of that test or any other scientific clinical test.

Surgery has no FDA (Spodick, 1975). Pills are expensively investigated by time-consuming, controlled, clinical tests before your doctor can prescribe them, but operations are not. Even with pills you must, of course, at last assume responsibility yourself, but you must be even more cautious before accepting an operation. Surgery lacks the quality control we might have expected it to have.

The reason is partly due to the great difficulty medical scientists have in testing operations with the "well controlled investigations" that the FDA requires for new drugs. If a controlled test seems necessary to evaluate an operation, the test calls for many patients willing to act as experimental subjects (only half of whom will have the operation being tested). The tests are expensive, last for years, and usually need the collaboration of investigators and patients from many medical centers (more about this in Chapter 18).

Should such an investigation of a surgical operation be carried out, it is subject to criticism on at least two major counts. First, the clinical test of an operation is almost never a "double-blind" test, as is the test of a new drug. A double-blind test requires that neither the doctor evaluating the results nor the patient undergoing the treatment knows which treatment was given—the new surgical operation under test in this instance, or its alternative, usually a medical treatment. When it comes to having had an operation or not, you can hardly fool anyone unless you perform a "sham" operation (the anesthesia, the incision, the whole works except for the definitive procedure under test) on those patients chosen, randomly, not to have the new operation (the controls). A sham operation is usually unacceptable, and its omission may diminish the value of a controlled test. I will, however, describe in Chapter 3 an instance when sham surgery was used effectively to discredit a useless operation.

The second major count on which to criticize large, controlled, surgical tests concerns a variable of no consequence in drug testing, but critical when testing surgery. That variable is the surgeon himself (Love, 1975). To put it simply: Surgeons are not as uniform as pills. A surgeon's skill and experience count and are often crucial to the success of the operation. The kind of person your surgeon is can make all the difference in an outcome. For this reason I devote an entire chapter (Chapter 20) to the matter of choosing a surgeon.

THE SURGEON

Surgeons vary in skill, experience, and personality, but the good ones all love to operate. Surgery is a great game. I have heard a famous American surgeon, chatting with a small group of slightly drunk fellow surgeons, say that he had come to believe that surgery was for the surgeon, not for the patient. Maybe he got this idea from Walt Whitman: "The oration is to the orator, the acting is to the actor and actress, not to the audience." No one spoke up to oppose this famous surgeon's point of view.

There is among many surgeons a certain confident swagger you might have noticed. An old story tells of three doctors—a general practitioner, an internist, and a surgeon—who went duck hunting. A bird appears. The GP says, "It looks like a duck, it flies like a duck, so I'm going to call it a duck." He blasts away and misses.

A second bird appears. It's the internist's turn. "It looks like a duck and flies like a duck," he says, "but we'll have to rule out the golden eagle and the whooping crane. They are endangered species, you know." Before he can fire a shot, the bird has flown over the horizon.

Now a third bird appears. The surgeon lifts his gun and fires. The bird drops at his feet. "Well, what do you know," he exclaims. "It's a duck!"

Few surgeons are this cavalier. Surgeons I've known care deeply and are very careful about what they are doing. But they sometimes have trouble establishing what's best; they don't know with adequate confidence when an operation is indicated. This may be because of what they don't yet know, or perhaps as Will Rogers said, "It's not what we don't know that causes trouble. It's what we know that ain't so."

GOOD OPERATIONS

At other times surgeons do know what's best. For accidents or emergencies an operation may be clearly indicated. A bleeding artery demands a ligature, a hole in the chest must be closed. Many congenital defects can be decisively corrected surgically.

When Cathy was four and had a head cold that didn't clear up, and then after that an earache, her mother took her to the family physician. He listened to her chest and heard a murmur of a kind he had heard before, but he wasn't absolutely sure about the diagnosis.

After he had treated her ear infection, he sent her to a cardiologist. "Typical," said this doctor to herself, "patent ductus arteriosus." Then she explained to Cathy's mother: "Cathy has an open channel between the two largest arteries as they leave the heart. It normally closes before birth. I think it can be fixed." The cardiologist explained how the enlarged heart was overworked and said that the defect, if untreated, would cause more trouble. Fortunately it could be completely cured by a relatively low-risk operation. Cathy had the operation. At the instant the duct was closed at surgery, her very next heartbeat became normal. She is now a physically normal young lady.

Many defects acquired over time and aging can also be surgically corrected.

A fifty-two-year-old surgeon noted one hot day, while wiping his face as he drove home, that he could not read the expressway exit-ramp signs with his left eye. After one quick look into that eye, his ophthalmologist made the diagnosis: cataract. Impossible! Wasn't he too young? But it was true. A change in glasses helped for a couple of months, but vision failed again, so the ophthalmologist removed the cataract, fitted a contact lens, and sight was restored—better than ever. Later the surgeon went through the same process with the right eye. His career as a surgeon—a person for whom keen sight is important—was saved.

The story is mine. Despite a surgeon's natural reluctance to have surgery performed on himself, I have, like many of us my age, had a couple of successful operations, plus one useless operation—a tonsillectomy at age five.

As with a cataract removal, the best operations are decisive. When the surgeon opens an obstructed intestine or unplugs a large artery, he may save a life. The best operations are anatomically and physiologically sound. They make sense even to one not learned in medical science. If a tumor appears, removal is reasonable. A hernia should be mended. If a gland produces too much hormone, perhaps part of that gland should be cut away.

Good operations are supported by scientific evidence. Often this comes down to the matter of the controlled testing that I mentioned above, but not always. Long-enduring, repeatedly confirmed usefulness, even without controlled testing, has established the value of a number of operations (hernia repair, for example). But this criterion can be tricky, since it may be confused with a surgical procedure's mere popularity.

Decisive success, where previously nothing else worked, has established other operations. A cancer of the lung had never been cured until a bold surgeon actually removed the diseased lung. It didn't require a controlled clinical test to confirm the patent-ductus-arteriosus operation that cured Cathy.

Nowadays a committee decision may propose to establish the usefulness of an operation. A Consensus Committee, usually appointed by some other committee, meets, and after long discussion, it defines the indications for a relatively new operation, such as kidney transplantation, say, or total hip replacement. The word of these seers is then passed by way of the medical literature down to the practicing doctors—possibly in lieu of substantial scientific evidence supporting the operation. These committees always seem to approve of the operation they are considering, probably because most of the members have a vested interest in it. They are chosen for the committee, as authorities, because they have experience using the operation, and of course they want to continue using it, so they approve it.

Surgery may always remain the best way to treat physical trauma, congenital defects (if they can't be prevented), and the mechanical effects of neglected or degenerative disease. The surgeon does his best work when he closes abnormal holes, relieves obstructions, excises local tumors, rebuilds body parts, and drains infections. In addition, surgery is still the best way to treat most cancers. The more recent innovations of major-organ transplantation, particularly of the kidney and heart, have been successful. Beyond these examples surgical innovators will always try to extend the craft, and sometimes they will succeed.

2

Operations to Avoid—
in Most Cases

The summer before he was to enter kindergarten, Tommy had a tonsillectomy. After a winter of head colds, his parents had decided they wanted no more of that. They had had tonsillectomies themselves before they entered school. Also, Tommy still wet the bed occasionally at night, especially after a busy day, and their doctor had told them of cases where, strange though it seemed, tonsillectomy had helped.

The night after his operation Tommy began to spit up a lot of blood. The nurses gave him a shot and applied cold packs to his neck, but before the bleeding stopped, Tommy aspirated some blood into his lungs. He ran a fever. When they took a chest X ray a few days later, it looked like pneumonia at first, but a pediatrician, who was called in, diagnosed a lung abscess. Antibiotics finally cleared the lung, but by then it was too late for Tommy to start school. He started a year later; by then he had stopped wetting the bed.

SIGNS OF UNNECESSARY SURGERY

In contrast to good operations, unnecessary operations, such as Tommy's, tend to be indecisive, physiologically unsound, and without adequate scientific support. A questionable operation may be recommended to you on faith rather than on evidence. "Trust me," says the surgeon, "it works well in my hands." Insist on more than that.

Your own judgment may tell you that the operation proposed for you just doesn't make good sense. If you find out that it is used more frequently in your city, in your town, or in your region of the country than in other places, beware. This may mean that its use depends on the number of eager surgeons available, rather than upon the number of needy patients. Styles of practice vary from place to place, but need is apt to be uniform.

Avoid operations for psychological disturbances that should be treated some other way. Surgeons can't really change sex. Also, on this basic level, surgery is the wrong way to treat obesity.

Refuse operations that alter function in order to treat complex diseases. (Stomach resection for chronic peptic ulcer is an example.) The physiologic principles justifying such operations are usually too intricate for straightforward surgical manipulation, and consequently the results are indecisive.

Turn down recommendations for an operation proposed to treat some aspect of a disease that's going to progress despite the operation. Surgery for widespread cancer is an example. For this same reason, be leery of operations used to treat degenerative diseases like atherosclerosis or arthritis. Surgery will not slow the general advance of such diseases. Atherosclerosis in a bypassed artery, as in coronary-artery surgery, may actually advance more rapidly after the bypass operation.

As with most guidelines, we can find exceptions to these. If advanced metastatic cancer causes intestinal obstruction or presses on nerves, surgery may prolong useful life and relieve pain. When the indications are sound, back surgery for degenerative changes in the spine will put many people back on their feet, uncomplaining. For morbid obesity—despite the fact that obesity may have a basic psychological origin not treatable surgically and that surgery may cause serious metabolic changes—surgery has lengthened undisciplined lives. Joint replacements for arthritis and vascular operations for atherosclerosis have at least partially restored physical vigor. It's even possible that an operation as discredited as brain lobotomy may have helped some psychiatric patients move out of the back wards before tranquilizers and thorazine came to dominate that kind of therapy.

Avoid operations for abnormalities that heal themselves. Small umbilical hernias in infants usually disappear, as do some apparently serious heart defects.

Maria, who had worked with me as a technician before she was married, called, on the verge of tears, to tell me that her firstborn child, a perfectly normal looking boy, had a heart murmur. The pediatricians had diagnosed a congenital ventricular septal defect (an abnormal opening between the lower heart chambers). That kind of defect may cause lifelong heart trouble and early death, Maria said, and she knew that it could be repaired by open-heart surgery, though there is a risk. What to do? Accept the risk of surgery?

No, wait. By the time Bobby was three, the murmur had disappeared; the defect had closed.

Almost half of ventricular septal defects in infants close spontaneously.

Don't expect too much of operations to relieve pain that has no precise, x-ray evident, anatomically identified cause; inadequately explained backache is an example of this kind of pain.

Most popular operations appear to make sense without the need of extensive testing. A time comes, say, when you don't really need your uterus any longer. Maybe it has some lumps (myomas) in it that the gynecologist says he can feel, or he points out that the uterus could become the site of a cancer someday. It's not doing you any good; let's take it out. Or if you have stones in your gallbladder, anyone can see that stones don't belong there. Get rid of them. When your child has a sore throat, the tonsils are always red and swollen, so why not have the tonsils out to prevent future attacks? If not the cause, the tonsils at least appear to be the focus of the disease. So it goes. These surgical solutions embody a roughshod kind of common sense, but the problems they propose to solve are complex, and surgery (which always carries a risk, even a fatal risk) may be an unreasonable solution to the problem—if there truly is a problem.

An operation that may at one time have appeared to make sense may finally have its irrationality exposed by additional research, experience, or recurring sanity.

ABANDONED OPERATIONS

Modern surgery, which started about a century ago when anesthesia and asepsis made it possible, has caught on wonderfully. We have over 20 million operations a year in this country, and many of these operations achieve marvelous benefits. Surgeons are justifiably proud of their record and talk about it. What they don't like to talk about are the operations they once performed and then abandoned because the operations were found to be useless or even harmful. Prominent surgeons enthusiastically recommended each of them. Thousands, even millions, of people submitted to some of them. In time, sometimes with the aid of scientific testing—and usually too slowly, at least when one looks back at the story—they were discredited. True, skeptical surgeons attacked use of the more outrageous examples from the beginning, but all of these operations had their staunch backers. Some were used by most of the surgical community for years. Perhaps knowing about these abandoned operations will sharpen your wariness of any modern operation that has been recommended for you. Is it one that may soon join this list?

Laparotomy, merely opening up the abdomen to expose the insides to air, was used to treat tuberculous peritonitis. It didn't make sense, but if it worked—what the hell! Surgeons told of their surprise and pleasure to find that it cured the disease. Anecdote supported it, not statistics. It really didn't work, of course, and sometimes things got worse, though it took a while to figure this out. It was abandoned even before antibiotics arrived to eliminate tuberculous peritonitis rationally.

The colon, located at the end of the intestine and the source of a fair amount of real trouble, has been accused by famous doctors, unjustly, of causing many troubles of which it is innocent. Maybe this is because it has always been linked, in fact and imagination, with the sewer; we are apt to think of it as a reservoir of poisons. Constipation—along with a slowed passage through the gut called stasis—allows poisons to accumulate and invade the system. Or so we have been told. Thus constipation causes "autointoxication" or acts as a "focus of infection."

If clysters and mineral oil didn't cure constipation, surgical elimination of the colonic reservoir itself would do the job. Surgeons have resected the colon for diseases as seemingly remote as epilepsy. "Run down" conditions or vague states of poor health, boredom, or apathy that once carried diagnoses such as "neurasthenia" or "chlorosis" ("greensickness")—and might be found these days under the spreading blanket of neurosis or emotional maladjustment—were attributed to the colon. During the early part of this century, Sir Arbuthnot Lane, a famous Scottish surgeon, built a reputation on surgery to bypass the colon and remove stasis (Gordon, 1983). He practiced with admirable technical skill. For most surgeons at that time colon surgery remained formidable and dangerous, and therefore—fortunately—Lane's operation never achieved wide currency. But tonsillectomy and tooth extraction to remove "focus of infection," carried out by lesser surgeons at the other end of the alimentary canal, did. They may still be so employed. What turns out to be the most obvious medical nonsense is sometimes hard to root out. (Though colectomy for stasis has passed from the scene, high-colonic-irrigation practitioners may still be found.)

Some years ago a cardiologist friend of mine, having suffered a small heart attack, confirmed by his own electrocardiograph, went all the way to the Cleveland Clinic, where surgeons freed up and tied off his internal mammary arteries and stuffed the stumps of these, now blind-ended, vessels into his heart's muscle. The needy heart was somehow expected to draw nourishment from these stumps. After an original flurry of interest in this operation a decade earlier, it had been abandoned, to be revived again, just before my friend had it, by the enthusiastic advocacy of a vocal Canadian surgeon who had found at last, he said, that the operation really worked—at least a little.

Then as now, surgeons needed something to do—anything. Appendectomy, always a staple of surgery, wasn't called for as often, and cancer of the stomach, curiously, had almost disappeared. A new pill that seemed to cure peptic ulcer better than surgery had come on the market. On top of this, internists were getting all of the business of the then booming heart-attack trade. Surgeons wanted to move in; they needed a new market.

My friend went back to full-time work after his operation and told me that he had evidence, on his electrocardiograph, that his heart had improved—a little. The operation had been worthwhile, he concluded. We didn't talk about how he might have been if he had just avoided the nonsense. In any case, this operation fell out of favor again rather promptly, but other operations, which he now recommends to his patients, judiciously, came along. He himself hasn't had one of the new ones. But he may; doctors, like members of high society, are apt to become the victims of fashion.

The operation this cardiologist had isn't the only operation once used for coronary artery disease but now abandoned. Ligation (closing off) of the internal mammary arteries (arteries that run down the chest wall just behind the breast bone), and something as silly, on the face of it, as shaking talcum powder into the sac that holds the heart (poudrage) were once popular, now abandoned, operations.

Since the early part of the century surgeons have targeted peptic ulcer—an open, nonhealing sore that usually appears in the first part of the small intestine, just beyond the stomach. They would treat this by connecting the stomach to the small intestine farther along, past the ulcer, thus taking the ulcer out of the food path (a gastroenterostomy). Or they might remove part of the stomach (to reduce the acid) and hook the remainder to the intestine beyond the ulcer (subtotal gastric resection).

A surgeon with whom I once worked had a subtotal gastric resection years ago. He says his ulcer doesn't bother him any more, but of course the removed part of his stomach never grew back. The remainder is so small that he has had to eat six times a day all these years, and he is as skinny as Ichabod Crane. He tends to eat alone at home—tiny meals, slowly.

Because gastroenterostomy was easier to perform than gastric resection and patients could still eat normal-sized meals in company, gastroenterostomy seemed to be winning the popularity contest a few decades ago. It kept operating rooms humming at some of our biggest clinics. Unfortunately, however, in the long run it didn't cure enough of the ulcers. It has been abandoned.

MY OWN RECORD

I trained on subtotal gastric resections, and I hated to quit. Once you learn how to do something like that moderately well, it's hard to give it up. But looking back now, I can see that neither of those operations for peptic ulcer were good operations. We never adequately tested them with controlled clinical studies that compared them with medical treatment; we just used them because they made sense to us, and at the time they seemed to work. They kept us busy. Drugs and better surgery have replaced them.

Gastric resections weren't my only mistakes of judgment. I've used a lot of subsequently abandoned operations. If the critical voice I have taken so far sounds like an effort to place myself above past surgical excesses, let me now confess: I've done my share of them. Just as I learned abdominal surgery doing gastric resections, I learned chest surgery doing another now abandoned operation, thoracoplasty (removal of ribs to collapse a lung infected with tuberculosis). Later, when surgery became a little more sophisticated and we had antibiotics to back us up, I resected the lung itself for tuberculosis; this turned out to be unnecessary because antibiotics alone would do the job. Then, not ready to give up on cutting into the lung for some damn reason or other, I resected parts of it for emphysema, truly a nonsurgical disease.

For cancer of the breast I used the superradical mastectomy—a bigger, more mutilating operation than the radical mastectomy—when the smart operators were beginning to use the lesser surgery that now dominates the field. For abdominal cancer I used "second looks" (repeated operations— as many as eight in one case) a kind of aggression that has been brought under more careful control by those who may still use it.

If this sounds as if I should have been disqualified years ago, hear my defense: I was traveling with a respectable crowd—my record not unusual. In its own way it epitomizes the history of modern surgery, and places me alongside those I am criticizing. Conscientious surgeons, among whom I count myself, have had a hard time learning how to justify an elective operation with convincing evidence. Modern, controlled, clinical testing may have improved the outlook, but surgery has been, and still is, often a guessing game.

THE SPECIALTIES, TOO

Every specialty of surgery has its abandoned operations. Brain lobotomy for psychiatric quandaries has been so widely condemned that we have all come to scorn it. In other regions of the nervous system, surgeons once removed the sympathetic nerves (nerves located along the spine) to treat high blood pressure, but they do so no longer.

Though not a neurosurgeon, George Crile, a famous surgeon of the first half of this century, was still taking out a collection of nerves from deep within the abdomen (the celiac ganglion) after, according to some of his competitors, he had gone blind (Crile, 1947). One of them, while visiting Crile's operating room, managed to get the specimen Crile had removed and have it examined by his own pathologist. It really was the celiac ganglion! Though his vision may have failed, Crile was still a master surgeon. But why, in the first place, did he remove the celiac ganglion? For high blood pressure, of course, to treat polyglandular disease, and possibly as a method of producing something called anoci-association (which no one has heard of for years). God knows!

Glands too—and particularly the adrenal gland—have been attacked surgically to treat high blood pressure. But probably no one ever matched the boldness of John R. Brinkley as a gland operator (Carson, 1960). In the 1920s and early 1930s, he transplanted goat testicles into the scrota of aging men to achieve sexual rejuvenation. Patients, whom he recruited by broadcasting his message over the most powerful radio station in the country, picked their own frisky donor goat and then submitted to a twenty-minute operation to restore their libido. After years of denunciation by more conservative members of the medical profession—and after he had finally abandoned the transplantation operation himself—Brinkley was discredited.

He is remembered as a blatant quack, though he did hold an M.D. degree (from a diploma mill) and an honorary degree from the Royal University of Pavia, Italy, and he had a license to practice medicine in several states. Perhaps his operation was more ridiculous than some of the other abandoned operations I am discussing; yet sometimes I find the borderline between quackery and establishment surgery a little indistinct.

Several other once popular operations on the urinary and genital systems have been abandoned. For instance, surgeons used to tack the kidneys back in position (nephropexy) for "floating kidney," and gynecologists have stitched the "tipped" womb into a posture they thought more proper in order to treat dysmenorrhea (painful menstruation). And so on and on. Other mature surgeons, like me, could provide their own lists of abandoned operations—records of mistakes, or at least of misguided good intentions, and a warning to you.

WARNING AND A LIST OF UNNECESSARY OPERATIONS

Your doctor will not have recommended a celiac ganglionectomy or a nephropexy for you, but the operation he has recommended could be an operation that will soon join this infamous list. History has a way of meddling with our present assurance, as George Santayana ("Those who do not know history are doomed to repeat it") and others have pointed out. We think we are more careful today than surgeons used to be. Perhaps we are, perhaps the "golden age" of surgery is past, and the specialty has become reliable, scientific, and humdrum—for the surgeon that is, not for the patient.

But surgery isn't flawless yet and may never be. Hindsight has guided my criticism of abandoned operations; foresight is precarious and controversial. Advocates will always find exceptions for their marginally useful operations on the basis of their experience, on anecdote, and on their prejudices. What I now believe is based on my experience, a reading of the medical literature, and common sense—I hope. Others will take exception, but I believe that in a significant percentage of the cases in which they are used, many modern operations are unnecessary. These include coronary-artery bypass grafting (CABG), percutaneous transluminal coronary angioplasty (PTCA), extra cranial-intracranial arterial bypass (EC-IC), hemorrhoidectomy, prostatectomy, cesarean section, hysterectomy, cholecystectomy, radial keratotomy for myopia, intervertebral disk surgery, tonsillectomy and adenoidectomy (T&A), circumcision, and middle ear ventilation. In the following chapters I'll explain why I think so.

John Kirklin, distinguished American surgeon, has provided this general warning: "Surgery is always second best. If you can do something else, it's better. Surgery is limited. It is operating on someone who has no place else to go."

In the last century Emily Dickinson wrote this:

> Surgeons must be very careful
> When they take the knife!
> Underneath their fine incisions
> Stirs the culprit—Life!

Finally, you, the patient, must decide whether an operation is necessary or not. To many, a mammoplasty following removal of the breast for cancer is unnecessary, but you, the patient, may regard it as essential. Try to become as well informed as you can before making your choice. If you choose surgery, you can usually find a compliant surgeon.

3

Coronary Artery Surgery

When his family doctor discovered an abnormal EKG on routine checkup, Henry Z., a thirty-nine-year-old New Jersey dentist, entered the hospital overnight for a catheterization that revealed narrowing of his coronary arteries. The doctor treated this condition with drugs, and Henry was able to do a full day's work with no symptoms except for one terrible side effect caused by the very drug that had stabilized his heart condition: No longer was he potent enough for sexual intercourse with either his wife, Carol, or his dental assistant, Wendy, who believed that she was somehow responsible for this startling change in Henry. She worked in the office after business hours with all her finesse to arouse him, but she failed.

The cardiologist had said, "Forget your heart now and live," but how could he "live" this way? He had a serious talk about surgery with the cardiologist, who then advised him further: "This operation is no picnic in the best of circumstances, and yours aren't the best. We even lose people, Henry. Live with it." A year of trying left Henry resentful and demoralized. He talked with his brother, the novelist Nathan Z., and finally decided to have the operation.

How did it come out? This story is from Phillip Roth's novel, *The Counterlife* (1986). In the novel the operation turns out more than one way, is performed on more than one character. It became a turning point in the story. Thus, we find that coronary-artery bypass grafting (CABG) has made a stunning entrance into fiction. In doing so, however, it and drugs as alternatives to the operation have been misrepresented. CABG has *not* been used as a way to cure sexual impotence. In fact, in one study, psychiatrists found that 57 percent of patients they interviewed were sexually impaired after surgery rather than improved. And beta-blocking drugs, such as propranolol, which may have been used to treat Henry, don't cause male impotency; it's a rare side effect.

If it hasn't often been used as a remedy for drug-induced sexual impotence, CABG has been used generously for the manifestations, or merely for the presence, of coronary artery disease. Much of the controversy that has surrounded the operation since its inception in 1967 has dealt with the indications for its use. Who needs it? CABG is a better operation than any of its numerous predecessors, and it helps some people, but it doesn't cure the disease. It is by no means ideal. Just the same it's very popular. At 280,000 a year, CABG has become one of the most frequent major operations done in this country.

Unfortunately, controlled clinical tests designed to determine sound indications for the operation—outcomes in surgical patients compared to those in patients treated medically—began only after surgeons were performing numerous operations on easily persuaded patients.

THE OPERATION

Because it requires elegant diagnostic methods, heart-lung bypass, and precise blood vessel surgery, CABG stands as a marvel of modern surgical accomplishment. Expensive facilities and specially trained teams now unite, in what some have called an industry, to carry out so many of these operations that their total cost consumes a considerable portion of our health-care expenses.

The medical system behind this operation may be complex, but the logic of the operation is simple. The two coronary arteries, right and left, supply blood to the heart itself. They are the first tributaries of the main artery (the aorta) just as it leaves the heart. Atherosclerosis of these arteries thickens their walls, and this thickening narrows the arterial channel, thereby reducing the blood flow to the heart. In cases where the narrowing is limited in extent and yet significant in degree, a blood vessel graft (a vein taken from the leg or a small artery taken from behind the breastbone) is connected during surgery to the main artery (the aorta), as it leaves the heart, and to the coronary artery beyond its narrow part, thus bypassing that part and bringing additional blood to the deprived muscle. The graft performs as an additional, or substitute, coronary artery.

In order to provide the surgeon with a quiet organ upon which to work, the patient's heart and lungs are bypassed during surgery by the heart-lung machine, which circulates the blood by means of a pump outside the body. The heartbeat is stopped. Although no heart chambers are opened, as they must be for certain congenital defects or for diseased valves, CABG is frequently spoken of as "open heart surgery."

If the graft remains open, the operation may succeed in strengthening the heart. On the other hand, the simple objective of the operation—to bring in new blood—may fail because the graft, often at the site where it is connected to the small artery, becomes obstructed. This is caused by technical failure or clotting due to the atherosclerosis. And arterial plugging may occur months or years after the operation as atherosclerosis advances, its nature tending to defeat the objectives of CABG. The operation in no way suspends the disease, which is usually widely dispersed in the coronary arteries at the time of surgery. Diffuse athero-sclerosis can be found when X rays have revealed only narrowing (McPherson et al., 1987).

Because of these uncertainties in the surgical management of this important disease (coronary heart disease, the leading cause of death in the United States, kills over 500,000 persons a year), medical scientists realized that they needed careful, scientific, clinical testing of the operation. Could the operation lengthen lives, or would it, on the average, endanger lives and waste money?

HISTORY

All earlier operations for coronary heart disease have been abandoned. CABG outclasses them because it makes more sense; it has a rational design. All but one of the earlier operations were taken up without controlled, clinical testing and given up only after something else came along. One operation, however, was subjected to rigorous, controlled, clinical testing of a kind that hasn't even been proposed for CABG, and when the testing demonstrated that the operation was useless, it was abandoned before many people had been victimized by it. Let's consider this old operation for a moment; we may learn something about appraising surgery, useful to present experience.

Thirty years ago surgeons advocated ligation of the internal mammary arteries (a relatively minor operation in which incisions are made on either side of the breast bone and arteries about an inch or so below the surface are simply tied off and cut across) as an effective treatment for angina (Beecher, 1961). Surgeons reported that 30 percent to 80 percent of their patients complained no more of angina. (Not much different from the reports currently published on the results of CABG, by the way.)

Two skeptical and independent surgical groups decided to test the operation with a double-blind study. Because it was a relatively safe and small operation, the control operations seemed justified. The patients agreed to the clinical test (informed consent). Half of them had their internal mammary arteries tied off, as the test operation, and the other half, as the controls, had only the skin incisions. None of the patients knew which operation they had undergone, test or control, nor did the evaluating physicians (thus, *double*-blind). It turned out that the control patients, who didn't have their internal mammary arteries ligated, had as much improvement as the test patients. After these findings were reported, surgeons abandoned this operation for angina.

We learn from this episode that surgery has a strong placebo effect. If an operation is done principally to reduce pain, about one third of the patients will report improvement due to a placebo effect. A placebo effect has been defined by S. Wolf (1959) as, "any effect attributable to a pill, potion, or procedure, but not to its pharmachodynamic or specific properties." In other words, though the effect is definite, its cause is not at all clear. Chemical processes in the brain seem to play a part. In any case, patients may improve after surgery whether or not the surgery brought about any significant anatomical or physiological alteration.

Since operations do produce this placebo effect, ideally many operations should be tested with double-blind clinical tests similar to the one used for internal mammary artery ligation. Both the control and the test patients, selected randomly, would have a surgical procedure: the control patients would have a sham operation (anesthesia, an incision, and so forth); only the test patients would have the actual anatomical alteration that is the essence of the operation under study. Neither the patients nor the evaluating physicians would know who was test and who was control, thus making it, as in the case of the internal-mammary-artery-test, a double-blind test.

Great idea! Works quite effectively for drug testing. It seems too much, however, in the name of science, to carry out a major operation, indistinguishable to the patient from a CABG, for example, at which, intentionally, nothing that might have helped was done. The controlled studies of CABG haven't gone that far, and hence they have failed to control the placebo effect of surgery. Nonetheless, they have made valuable comparisons of CABG with medical treatment (which, understandably, has its own placebo effect).

CLINICAL TESTING

The first large controlled study (Veterans Administration trial) showed relatively little benefit from the operation except in a small subgroup of patients (Murphy et al., 1977), but it did nothing to dampen enthusiasm for the operation. Advocates believed that new scientific studies would provide better results, thus scientifically underpinning their enthusiasm (and profit), so new studies were started in this country and in Europe, at great expense. After three major studies had been carried out—the Veterans Administration Cooperative Study (VA trial), the European Coronary Surgery Study (ECSS 1982), and the Coronary Artery Surgery Study (CASS 1983)—the main questions to be answered were: Does bypass surgery prolong life? Does it affect the rate of subsequent heart attacks? Are there patients with certain kinds of coronary artery disease who may be uniquely benefited?

INDICATIONS

Because of the popularity and the large profit-making potential of this operation, explications of the results of these studies—to rival the exegeses of theologians when contemplating the Dead Sea Scrolls—have appeared and doubtless will continue to appear, but the important, and relatively unbiased, conclusions seem to be as follows (Braunwald, 1983):

1. Bypass surgery improves survival in patients with significant obstruction of the left main coronary artery. (There are left and right coronary arteries. The left main coronary artery divides into two branches: circumflex and anterior descending. "Significant obstruction" usually means at least a 50 percent reduction in the diameter of the artery, as determined by preoperative, angiograph X rays.)

Patients with significant obstruction of the left main coronary artery have usually made up less than 10 percent of candidates for surgery.

2. Bypass surgery appears to improve survival in high-risk patients with three-vessel disease (significant obstruction of the circumflex, the left anterior descending, and the right coronary arteries) plus measurably reduced pumping capacity of the heart. Although patients with unstable angina (increasing severity of the angina) have a similar outcome whether they receive medical therapy alone or coronary bypass surgery plus medical therapy, a subgroup of these with reduced pumping capacity of the heart may have a better two-year survival rate after coronary bypass (Luchi et al., 1987).

3. Bypass surgery does not protect from the risk of subsequent heart attacks.

4. The graft tends to close in time (particularly if the graft is a vein), and the bypassed artery may develop atherosclerosis at an increased rate.

5. The overall six-year survival rate for surgical patients in the CASS (large controlled United States study) was 92 percent and for medical patients 90 percent (Kolata, 1983). Thus, patients who are functioning well do not need bypass unless they have the high-risk conditions mentioned under 1 and 2.

6. If there are no contraindications, patients with angina unrelieved by medical treatment are candidates for CABG. In fact, the operation has worked best in the relief of angina. But remember the example I gave above. Ligation of the internal mammary arteries—an operation that was discredited thirty years ago after a double-blind, random-controlled study—also relieved angina: a result of surgery's placebo effect.

Inasmuch as the operation won't prolong life or prevent further heart attacks for most candidates, doctors are left with something called an improved "quality of life." They recommend surgery for that. The operation will make you feel better, they say; you'll have less angina, and you'll lead a more active life. When interviewed after surgery, many patients attest to these benefits, but the CASS study showed no difference between operated and nonoperated groups in the amount or type of recreational activity and no difference in the numbers who returned to work. Moreover, angina gradually worsened with time in both groups.

Paul Meir, a statistician who studied the CASS data, said (Kolata, 1981): "What we offer patients is not a longer life but a different perception of themselves—a return to normal. Medical patients have no reason to deny their symptoms. But we must weigh reports of a patient's symptoms after surgery with the patient's belief that he has now done the maximum possible for his disease." Meir also noted that one way to interpret the finding that a large number of surgical patients do not return to work "is as a devastating comment on the claim of improvement in life-style."

Psychiatrists, who studied a small group of patients one to two years after surgery, found that 83 percent were unemployed and 57 percent were sexually impaired (Gundle 1980). Most patients who had suffered angina eight months or longer evidenced a damaged self-concept, they said, which was reinforced rather than repaired by the experience of surgery.

Angina, as I said, has been a principal indication for CABG, and postoperatively many patients say they are relieved of this symptom, but a lot of odd, subsequently abandoned therapies have relieved angina (Benson and McCallie, 1979): heart muscle extract, pancreatic extract, various hormones, xanthines, khellin, x-ray irradiation, anticoagulants, monoamine oxidase inhibitors, thyroidectomy, radioactive iodine, sympathectomy, various vitamins, choline, meprobamate, ligation of the internal mammary arteries (discussed above), epicardial abrasions, and cobra venom.

ALTERNATIVES

The operation remains more popular than one would expect. In commenting on this, Vallee Willman, a surgeon who served on a Consensus Panel studying the data, said (Kolata, 1981): "It is difficult for physicians to spend time to medically manage patients and encourage changes in life-style. It is easier to encourage surgery . . . The patients want the consolation of having done everything possible. Surgery is at least a tangible assault on the process."

The changes in life-style that Dr. Willman refers to—more exercise, no smoking, low-fat, low-cholesterol diet—have enlisted the advocacy of prestigious committees as well as the American Heart Association. We are becoming a nation of soft-vegetarians (perhaps a bit of chicken and fish with the veggies), street runners, and health-club activists. All to the good.

In a report to the American Heart Association, measurable widening of the arteries was found in a small group of patients put on a low-fat, vegetarian diet, in which less than 10 percent of calories were from fat, mostly unsaturated (Ornish et al., 1988). The patients also received an exercise program and stress-management training, including yoga and meditation. No smoking.

Said Alexander Leaf, one of the project directors: "It's extremely important to show that without drugs, just by changing people's life-style, you can get coronary-artery disease to regress." In another recent study various kinds of induced mental stress were shown to produce abnormalities indicating reduced blood flow to the heart (Rozanski et al., 1988). So, relax. Maybe a change in life-style should start early. A New York study of fourth- to eighth-graders found that blood cholesterol, an important risk factor for coronary heart disease, was lowered after an educational program focusing on diet, physical activity, and nonsmoking (Walter et al., 1988).

I endorse the movement; I have been running for years, and I haven't eaten butter since the 1950s, when this idea first surfaced, as I remember, in a book titled: *Eat Well and Stay Well* (Keys, 1959), one of the first in a deluge of low-fat diet books.

Cardiologists have been speaking up more lately to recommend new drugs based on sound pharmacology. Following an embarrassing history of many abandoned drugs for angina, medical scientists have at last come up with some effective drugs (Plotnick, 1978; Braunwald, 1983; Luchi, et al., 1987). Beta-adrenergic blockers (propranolol, trade name Inderal, for example) improve survival in patients who have had heart attacks, and they lower blood pressure. Drugs called calcium-channel blockers improve the outlook in certain kinds of angina where the vessels may be going into spasm. The treatment of even mild high blood pressure helps. Sometimes digitalis for heart failure or drugs to treat irregular heartbeat are required. Nitroglycerin still works, and common aspirin improves survival in some types of angina (Aspirin, 1980). As the CASS study showed, pills may help as much as surgery. Maybe neither is required.

Clot-dissolving drugs have made a big splash. Though not clear alternatives to CABG, because CABG is most often employed for chronic complaints, these drugs have become crucial in treating acute heart attacks—nearly three quarters of a million each year in the United States. By dissolving the clot that causes a heart attack and thus opening the blocked coronary artery, they may conceivably forestall a later need for CABG. Prompt use of these drugs lowers heart-attack mortality by as much as 40 percent, but there is debate as to whether TPA (tissue plasminogen activator), a new entry, is better than streptokinase, longer on the scene and much cheaper. Good evidence suggests that they have similar effects (White, 1989). Furthermore, a new drug, APSAC (anisoylated plasminogen streptokinase activator complex) (Rapaport, 1989), is yet to be compared with the other two in controlled tests.

TPA, manufactured by Genentech using recombinant DNA technology, made pharmaceutical history by racking up $93 million in sales, at $2,200 per treatment, in the first four months of its sale. It's the fastest-selling new drug in history. Complicating TPA's introduction have been allegations of a possible conflict of interest involving at least thirteen members of the study group responsible for its clinical testing, who held stock or stock options in Genentech (Marx, 1988).

I'll describe the use of these clot-dissolving drugs along with PTCA (percutaneous transluminal coronary angioplasty) in the next chapter. There, too, controversy prevails.

Eugene Braunwald, prominent cardiologist and medical educator, said in 1983 that he thought a combination of factors would arrest the growth of CABG surgery and possibly cause a decline in its frequency: (1) the improved effectiveness of nonsurgical treatment and possibly greater use of coronary angioplasty (to be discussed in the next chapter); (2) the lack of statistical evidence in the CASS study that survival is improved in any other than those patients with disease of the left main coronary artery (see above); (3) increasing efforts to contain the costs of medical care, especially of procedures whose indications have not been clearly established; and (4) a continued decline in the incidence of coronary-artery disease.

Indeed, deaths due to coronary-artery disease *have* fallen since about 1967 when CABG was first used (Gomez-Marin et al., 1987), but this cannot be attributed to CABG or to any treatment administered by doctors. As with the decreased incidence of cancer of the stomach, it is one of those surprising and gratifying improvements in health that can likely be credited to a general change in diet or a general change in our pattern of living, not to the direct intervention of the practicing medical establishment.

CURRENT USE, EFFORTS AT CONTROL

Despite predictions that after the CASS report, surgeons would use it less, the frequency of CABG increased from 202,000 operations in 1984 to 282,000 in 1986 (last year for data). How many of these expensive operations are unneeded? Some guess the number to be 25,000 to 30,000

(*Medical Journal Bulletins*, 1987); I would suspect it's a lot more than that.

In what manner *is* CABG being used? A 1988 study from UCLA and the Rand corporation suggests it is used inappropriately (Winslow et al., 1988a). They conclude that surgeons frequently ignore sound indications for the operation; they perform a large number of unneeded CABGs. After sorting out the best indications—from among 488 possible indications—with a national panel of presumed experts, the investigators compared these with actual practice in 386 cases at three randomly chosen hospitals. By their criteria 56 percent of the surgeries were performed for appropriate reasons, 30 percent for equivocal reasons, and 14 percent for inappropriate reasons. The percentage of appropriate surgeries varied, hospital-to-hospital, from 37 percent to 78 percent.

You might avoid falling into the wrong percentage by seeking a second opinion. What happens then? Researchers at Harvard evaluated eighty-eight persons who had been referred for a second opinion after a first opinion recommended CABG (Graboys, 1987). The cardiologists who gave the second opinion advised continuation of medical treatment in seventy-four cases (84 percent). Sixty of the seventy-four chose this option; the remaining fourteen had surgery sooner or later. During a two-year follow-up, none died and only four—two in each group—had heart attacks. Conclusions: Second opinions for motivated patients provide a safe option. Most patients will adhere to a second opinion recommending medical treatment, thus reducing the need for surgical intervention by as much as 50 percent. Half of CABG operations may be unnecessary!

Regardless of frequent assertions in medical and lay publications that bypass surgery was overused, business boomed, and analysts, granting that the randomized clinical trial is still the best test, found encouragement in their uncontrolled studies (Califf et al., 1989). Now, however, growth has slackened. The advent of percutaneous transluminal coronary angioplasty (PTCA) has stolen many promising cases (see next chapter) and for many a cardiac surgeon oversupply brings with it a struggle to maintain, or achieve, a respectable caseload. Surgeons fear that without a certain volume, which will probably settle out at about 200 CABG operations a year, they may lose out altogether. Third-party players, including Medicare, may decide to refuse compensation for low-volume operators.

This prospect follows from evidence that hospitals and surgical teams that perform more than 200 CABG operations per year have fewer patient deaths, shorter lengths of stay, and lower charges (Dateline, 1987). One study concluded that "the greatest improvement in average outcomes for CABG surgery would result from the closure of low-volume surgery units" (Showstack et al., 1987). Perhaps, say some authorities, cardiac services should be regionalized—not likely, however, without a major health-service revision. Another study estimated that thirty-seven deaths following bypass surgery could be avoided for every 1,000 patients transferred from hospitals performing 215 or fewer procedures per year, to hospitals performing more than 215 per year—the cutoff point of 215 chosen empirically (Robinson et al., 1987).

To you this may mean that if, despite what you have read so far, you still plan to consider the operation, you should select a place with a large volume. Experience counts. Be especially vigilant about choosing a hospital at near the 200-per-year level, however. These operators, aware that they are going to have to continue breaking the 200 level each year, may work too hard to sell their product—use more generous indications for the operation, perform more needless operations than a 500-per-year outfit, which can afford more stringent indications and still handily break the caseload limit.

You might consider going to one of the centers that participated in the CASS* investigation for evaluation, or perhaps for a second opinion after a local recommendation. Physicians at these centers might, at the very least, be expected to follow the approved indications.

* Clinical Centers participating in CASS with principal investigators: University of Alabama, Birmingham, William J. Rogers, M.D.; Albany Medical College of Union University, Albany N.Y., Eric D. Foster, M.D.; Boston University Medical Center and Evans Memorial Department of Clinical Research, Boston, Thomas J. Ryan, M.D.; Loma Linda University School of Medicine, Loma Linda, Calif., C. Joan Coggin, M.D.; Marshfield Medical Foundation, Inc., Marshfield Clinic, Marshfield, Wis., William O. Myers, M.D.; Massachusetts General Hospital, Boston, J. Warren Harthorne, M.D.; Mayo Clinic, Rochester, Minn., Robert L. Frye, M.D.; Miami Heart Institute, Miami Beach, Fla., Arthur J. Gosselin, M.D.; Institut de Cardiologie de Montreal, Montreal, Martial G. Bourassa, M.D.; New York University Medical Center, New York, Ephraim Glassman, M.D.; St. Louis University School of Medicine, St. Louis, George C. Kaiser, M.D.; St. Luke's–Roosevelt Hospital Center, New York, Harvey G. Kemp, M.D.; Stanford University Medical Center, Stanford, Calif., Edwin L. Alderman, M.D.; The Medical College of Wisconsin, Veterans Administration Medical Center, Milwaukee, Harold R. Brooks, M.D.; Yale University School of Medicine, New Haven, Conn., Lawrence S. Cohen, M.D.

4

More Blood Vessel Surgery

PTCA—Percutaneous Transluminal Coronary Angioplasty

"Bill, why are you sleeping so much?" complained his wife, Ann. "The lawn has to be mowed, and what'll the neighbors think?"

Bill sat up on the couch and shrugged. "I don't feel like it." He hadn't felt like doing much of anything for some time now—a nagging discomfort in his chest stopped him when he hurried.

Finally, at Ann's insistence he went to see a doctor, who found an abnormality in his electrocardiograph, more evident when Bill did an exercise test. "Your blood pressure is high, Bill, and these changes in the EKG mean that your heart isn't up to snuff. I'll start you on some beta blockers for your blood pressure, but I think you ought to have an X ray of your coronary arteries. Maybe something can be done."

Bill hated the idea of surgery or anything radical, but this sounded okay. He knew something was wrong, so why not get at the cause? His doctor referred Bill to Dr. Perkins, a cardiologist who had just returned from an intensive course on PTCA (percutaneous transluminal coronary angioplasty), the new way of splitting open narrowed coronary arteries. Dr. Perkins admitted Billy to the hospital, where they x-rayed his coronary arteries (coronary angiogram). Just as they placed the catheter in the left coronary artery, Bill's heart skipped a couple of beats, then speeded up. For a minute Dr. Perkins thought that the heart might go into ventricular fibrillation (fatal irregularity if uncorrected), but after intravenous medication, it beat regularly; they completed the examination.

"There are a couple of regions in your coronary arteries that are narrow," explained Dr. Perkins, "but the good news is that it's the kind of narrowing we can get at. We might follow you, see what happens to your symptoms when your blood pressure has been down for a while, but I think you might as well have the arteries opened up. They won't open up by themselves, you know."

"You mean an operation? What do you call it? A bypass? Gosh!" Bill felt his face flush; his pulse jumped. "I don't know."

"No, this would be easier to take than a coronary bypass operation. We put a little tube in the artery, much like the catheter we used for the x-ray pictures, but this catheter has a tiny balloon on the end. When the balloon is in the narrow part we inflate it, under careful control, of course. That opens up the narrowed artery so more blood reaches your heart where it's needed."

"You mean not an operation? But what if something happens?"

"If we really need them, the coronary bypass team will be standing by, but we don't need them very often."

Bill shook his head. "Gosh, I don't know. This is sort of sudden. I'll have to talk it over with my wife."

When they talked it over, Ann asked, "Don't you think you should get a second opinion, or at least wait a while, maybe go someplace else where you're sure they have done a lot of these . . . whatever-you-call-em?"

"Angioplasty . . . or PTCA, that's what they call them. I just don't know, but I'd sure like to get this thing over with and get back to normal."

"Does the operation cure your condition?"

"Well, I don't know for sure, but it opens up the artery. Apparently that's what I need."

A week later Bill had an angioplasty of one of the two narrowed branches of his coronary arteries. Dr. Perkins thought that would be enough. After all, he had done only eighteen of these on his own, and he didn't want to start getting into trouble.

Two weeks after the angioplasty Bill was feeling better than he had for weeks. He started to take short, brisk walks every day and promised Ann that he would soon give up smoking altogether and lose a little weight. Ann said that she intended to take a course on low-fat cooking.

To the dismay of heart surgeons, who can't do much about it, PTCA has invaded the terrain of CABG. The cardiologist or roentgenologist, skilled at passing a tiny catheter into the coronary arteries through which he injects a dye that shows up on X ray, uses a similar catheter with a balloon for PTCA. After he passes the ballooned catheter upward through an artery in the thigh and then into the coronary arteries, he locates the balloon in the narrowed part (if possible), and inflated it to enlarge the artery. Downgraded to a standby crew, the proud surgical team waits in case they are needed—if, for example, the cardiologist fouls up.

But of course the diseased artery may not cooperate, the technique is difficult, and the catheters are complex. They have to reach a precise location, and after doing their job, slip out easily. Over the years catheters with balloons near their ends have become smaller, more intricate, and more widely useful. The evolution of ballooned catheters started in the 1930s with Foley, a St. Paul, Minnesota, urologist, who, with his dining-room table as workbench, vulcanized rubber balloons to the ends of urinary catheters. A Foley catheter in the urinary bladder with its balloon inflated would remain there until the balloon was deflated or broken. Every doctor has used Foley's invention, and Foley, leaving the workbench behind, became a rather elegant man. I remember him, preceded by a private chauffeur carrying the doctor's lecture materials, when he appeared before us awed junior medical students. Would we ever have chauffeurs? No way.

Thomas Fogarty, a Cincinnati surgeon at the time, attached smaller balloons to smaller catheters and entered blood vessels to clean out clots successfully (Fogarty et al., 1963). This technique, too, has become firmly established in the medical armamentarium. Next, an Oregon radiologist, Charles Dotter, while taking x-ray pictures of arteries narrowed by atherosclerosis, conceived of new uses for catheters with little balloons (Annexton, 1978). Reporting on his work in 1963, Dotter said, "I am convinced that the relief of atheromatous obstruction in small arteries can best, perhaps only, be accomplished by means of catheter techniques. . . ." He used his catheters to open up narrowed arteries in the thigh, thus contributing Percutaneous Transluminal Angioplasty

(PTA) as an alternative to the direct scraping out or the bypassing of leg arteries, as done by vascular surgeons.

But vascular surgeons were skeptical; a surgeon's objective has always been to see what he is about—open surgery—usually at some price. Open-heart surgery, as an example, required more complex, demanding, and expensive techniques than closed operations, but it won out because the surgeon could see what he was doing. Dotter's closed PTA technique gained acceptance slowly in this country; it made more progress in Europe.

The coronary arteries, much smaller, more tortuous, and more difficult to enter, became accessible to Dotter's technique with the better catheters and guiding tools devised by Andreas Grüntzig of Zürich, Switzerland, who brought PTCA on the scene (1979), a technique now continually modified by a confusing array of variations and "improvements." Best estimates are that at least 200,000 of these procedures were performed in 1986. No wonder that the cardiac surgeon fears a loss of trade, or at least a fading of his growth industry.

Forget the poor surgeon. With PTCA, you, as a patient, might escape the chest operation, the heart-lung machine, the precarious graft, and all the paraphernalia of CABG. Sounds reasonable. But the picture is still blurred. Maybe you don't need either PTCA or CABG, and if you need something, your doctor may not really know what you need. Or perhaps you could try first one and then, if needed, the other? That's being done too. The whole endeavor sounds a little frantic at times with "salvage" PTCAs, emergency CABGs, etc. It's a mixture of marvelous technique and uncertain application.

While cardiologists hurry to acquire enough experience—on willing subjects—to become slick operators, and while they purchase the latest instruments (enthusiastically pushed by instrument makers), they justify the procedure by assuming that PTCA will achieve effects similar to CABG (Bredlau, 1985). Indications are the same, they say, but they have little evidence that indications *are* the same, and they haven't used PTCA for the same kinds of cases. They regularly extend its use beyond sound clinical indications for CABG (see Chapter 3), but avoid using it for multiple narrowings. Most candidates for PTCA have had single-vessel disease, but there aren't many indications for CABG in single-vessel disease unless the single vessel is the left main coronary artery—an artery for which PTCA is usually not employed.

Early, the National Heart, Lung, and Blood Institute established a voluntary registry of cases undergoing this procedure (the NHLBI PTCA Registry)—not a controlled test such as I have discussed in Chapter 3, but at least a central listing of cases (Mock, 1984). They tried to give some semblance of order and concern to the explosive use of this new and untested procedure. By 1984 they reported on 3,079 cases in the registry (obviously only a tiny fraction of the cases actually done). This report and a second extension of the study on 1,802 patients, reported in 1988, provided the best data on the results and status of PTCA (Detre et al.).

Mortality rate was 0.9 percent in the first study and 1 percent in the second, in which patients were older with more widespread disease; 5 percent and 4.3 percent, respectively had heart attacks brought on by the procedure. The need for emergency CABG during the angioplasty hospitalization dropped from 6.6 percent in the first to 3.9 percent in the second study, and the overall success rate increased from 61 percent to 78 percent. Tests of heart muscle blood supply in the first study, however, showed that it was about the same before and after PTCA. A recurrence of the arterial narrowing (restenosis) occurred in 7 percent (others say as high as one third have restenosis). Although most (84 percent) of the successful cases reported angina relief, no more of them went back to work after the procedure. Average dollar-saving per PTCA, compared with CABG cost, was $7,149. Said the author of a summary (Mock, 1984): "There are still many unanswered questions concerning the relative merits of PTCA and CABG in treating patients with CAD (coronary heart disease). In addition, restenosis remains a significant problem." Long-term efficacy of current angioplasty remains to be determined, said the investigators.

In summary, these figures mean that, fortunately, the mortality rate for the procedure is low, that relatively few patients are seriously damaged by it, and that most feel better after they have it. But we still don't know for what cases it's better than medical treatment or better than CABG. It has, nonetheless, been accepted as the preferred technique for narrowing of a single coronary artery, limited in extent, and it's being used more often for multivessel disease (stenosis in more than one blood vessel) (Kent, 1987). Practitioners, at least those in the NHLBI registry, are acquiring more skill. No controlled, randomized clinical trials concerning its general use—the essential test for this type of procedure—have been reported, but an important trial of its use following heart attack has been reported (see below).

In a summary of the 1984 report on the Registry one commentator said

(Willman, 1984), "Many investigators fully endorse a prospective clinical randomized trial and believe that in the absence of such information, clinical practice will be on uncertain footing." Why then no randomized clinical trial on its general use? One reason seems to be that authorities recognize that unless investigators could study very large numbers of patients, the trials probably wouldn't show a significant difference between the various treatment styles.

So PTCA remains on "uncertain footing" while more and more patients submit, and its advocates lack the evidence a clinical trial might provide. Advocates of PTCA and CABG have not endorsed such trials. What troubles them, I think, is that the mortality rate is low and angina relief high for patients in all the groups (medically treated, CABG, and PTCA); therefore, a clinical trial would not likely detect significant differences among these alternatives. As in the case of the clinical trials that compared medical treatment and CABG, the differences, if they did appear, probably wouldn't be great. In short, it probably wouldn't make much difference whether you have the procedure or not.

Before investigators can get organized and carry out a sound clinical test of PTCA—if they are so inclined—something else will surely come along. They will soon be testing an obsolete operation, their procedure replaced by something new. Laser angioplasty keeps making the news, and it has reached application in peripheral vascular disease (Gunby, 1987). (Anything with "laser" in it has been a fairly good bet.) Stainless steel tubes of mesh or wire are being fitted into the artery to hold it open (Sigwart et al., 1987; Goldsmith, 1988), and others have devised an ingenious device actually to scrape out the gunk lining the vessels (Kirn, 1989). More is sure to appear.

Surgeons have lost the turf battle that has awarded PTCA to the cardiologists, or radiologists. Earlier, as diagnosticians, cardiologists had taken up cardiac catheterization (invented by a surgeon, as a matter of fact), first for the right side of the heart, and then, with a more challenging technique, for the left side. Coronary angiograms, which require that a small catheter be passed upstream in a thigh artery to reach the heart and then out into the arteries of the heart (the coronary arteries), came next. By injecting a dye that can be seen on X ray, they could, with previously unknown precision, diagnose the extent and degree of coronary atherosclerosis. Next, with the still more challenging technique of PTCA, they could place a balloon in the narrowed artery, dilate it, and thus treat the disease they had diagnosed.

Previously, only diagnosis had been in the hands of internists and radiologists; now nonsurgeons, who at the beginnings of their careers had shown neither special aptitude nor interest in technique per se, were using an elegant and complex new technique—this an interesting, and at times turbulent, shift in the nature of specialization. Surgeons still control admission to the operating room, but these nonsurgeons have bypassed the operating room and, though with no conspiracy in mind, come to dominate an important new invasive technique.

Two-day training programs have sprung up, to which practitioners flock, there learning how to insert and control the newest gadgets without mauling the coronary arteries dangerously. The balloon, investigators have learned, doesn't just stretch the artery, it splits the plaque of atherosclerotic material that has caused the narrowing (Block, 1984). This leaves a rough-edge wound in the vessel wall; its healing process, they say, poorly understood. More study needed, and better technology, too.

In the search for better technology, a competition among surgeons, cardiologists, and radiologists—described as the Vascular War of 1988— this time for peripheral-vascular-surgery rather than heart-surgery patients, has heated up (Zarins, 1989; Wexler et al., 1989). Previously, medical care as well as surgical intervention in patients with leg-vessel atherosclerosis (peripheral vascular disease) fell to vascular surgeons. Then Dotter (see above), a radiologist, came along with his balloon angioplasty, but his technique, applied only infrequently by vascular surgeons, who were still in control, didn't disseminate as well here as it did in Europe. In Europe Grüntzig, a cardiologist, applied Dotter's technique to the heart (PTCA).

Following his bold attack, many nonsurgeons soon invaded the blood-vessel surgery terrain. In peripheral vascular cases (narrowing of blood vessels in the extremities) they find that they can test new techniques such as laser angioplasty before they apply them to the field of the coronaries—potentially more lucrative, but technically more challenging and more dangerous. Leg arteries, being larger than coronaries, are easier to work with—failure is less catastrophic. As a result of their successful invasion of the peripheral-vascular territory, nonsurgeons have discovered new opportunities for angioplasty and may now be found treating arterial lesions that vascular surgeons wouldn't have touched with their old techniques. These new interventions are undertaken without clinical testing or any evidence that such intervention helps.

Hold off if you can. Delay may pay off for you. In PTCA we have, once again, a popular, not very effective, halfway technology with ill-defined indications. You could end up with an obstructed coronary artery that originally was only narrow, or with one that is widened a little, but only briefly. PTCA is improving; already it seems better and safer than CABG for many patients. And something new may arrive to outclass these palliative operations, perhaps even something that is in some way actually curative.

Alternatives are the same as they are for CABG—pills, exercise, no smoking, good hygiene, etc. See Chapter 3.

PTCA FOR HEART ATTACKS

PTCA's advocates have employed the technique as an emergency operation—enthusiastically but not always wisely. If it's a heart attack that inspires your doctor to recommend a PTCA, you may feel that the emergency allows little choice—you have to go along. Instead, prepare yourself to make an informed decision, whether for yourself or for someone who asks your help. Hold to the slightly detached, mildly amused, attitude I hope you have by now adopted toward this medical bedlam.

No amusement is to be found in the fact that about 1.5 million Americans suffer heart attacks each year. This somber story is relieved, however, by some good news: Because of decreased incidence and improved survival from heart attacks, mortality from coronary heart disease has fallen 40 percent in the last two decades (Gomez-Marin, 1987). Neither doctor's office nor general hospital care has caused the decrease, but treatment in intensive care units may have contributed to it. More recently thrombolytic (clot-dissolving) drugs (see Chapter 3) have transformed care; they promise to improve survival further. Formerly, heart-attack treatment was passive, now it has become aggressive— sometimes, it appears from recent reports, too aggressive.

A thrombolytic drug—often TPA, but perhaps more frequently strep-tokinase, since it appears to be as effective and is cheaper (White et al., 1989)—is given immediately, within four hours of the heart attack if possible. Then, in what has been called a blitzkrieg strategy, the patient undergoes a coronary angiogram (X ray of the artery), this to be followed by an immediate PTCA if the X rays show any remaining obstruction in the involved artery (Cheitlin, 1988). Controlled studies have established the value of thrombolytic drugs, but not that of immediate angiography and PTCA.

A report from the Thrombolysis in Myocardial Infarction (TIMI) Research Group, designed to assess the role of PTCA after thrombolysis with TPA, describes results with two groups: a group subjected to angiography and prophylactic PTCA immediately and a delayed group not subjected to this blitzkrieg. No difference was found in most factors considered important, and more complications turned up in the PTCA group (TIMI Research Group, 1988). A second report (TIMI Research Group, 1989) focused on the delayed group, who were subjected to angiography and PTCA, if the vessels were suitable, eighteen to forty-eight hours after TPA. It concludes: "In patients with acute myocardial infarction [heart attack] who were treated with rt-PA [TPA] and heparin followed by aspirin, an invasive strategy of coronary arteriography 18 to 48 hours after the onset of symptoms, followed by prophylactic PTCA, offered no advantage. . . ." PTCA for heart attack victims failed to reduce the rate of subsequent trouble.

The blitzkrieg strategy has been discredited, but once again, only after it had become a rather common practice. Other studies reached similar conclusions (Topol et al., 1987: Guerci et al., 1987). Immediate use of the thrombolytic drugs is justified but not immediate catheterization with the intent of possible PTCA. CABG? Its role, if any, after thrombolytic drugs was not defined by these studies.

Thomas Graboys (1989) has pointed out the strong financial interest that hospitals have in cardiovascular surgery and angioplasty programs. The competition is intense, and they counsel one another to have a strategy of "keeping the funnel full." You, I think, should try to avoid being sucked into that funnel.

ARTERIES TO THE BRAIN

Hardening (atherosclerosis) attacks all arteries, not only the arteries of the heart. With special devastation it attacks arteries supplying the brain, resulting in stroke, which appears in 750,000 new cases a year. Stroke kills a quarter of a million persons in the United States every year (ranked third as a cause of death, behind heart disease and cancer)—and its usual mechanism is obstruction or rupture of a diseased artery. A surgeon's logic tells him then, that if a critical artery to the brain is narrowed because of atherosclerosis, thus forecasting obstruction and stroke, the artery should be surgically opened or bypassed to avert catastrophe.

Two surgical measures have been designed on the basis of this logic. One, to open a major artery in the neck if it is narrowed or obstructed—carotid endarterectomy—two, to bypass an obstruction within the cranium—extracranial-intracranial arterial bypass (EC-IC). Success with the first has generally been good, though it is probably overused. The second, a more recent invention, though ingenious and the subject of much study, appears now to be ineffective. If your doctor recommends EC-IC, I think you may decide, from the following account, to say no.

EXTRACRANIAL-INTRACRANIAL
ARTERIAL BYPASS (EC-IC)

Success with microvascular surgery in the extremities encouraged neurosurgeons to operate on small arteries supplying the brain. In 1965 surgeons in Nara, Japan, first reimplanted a finger by reconnecting tiny arteries and veins that are no more than a millimeter or two in diameter. This demanding technique still finds its widest and most gratifying application for reimplanting digits, but success here stimulated surgeons to extend small-vessel surgery to slightly larger diseased vessels. If they could reconnect the tiny vessels of a finger, maybe they could work with atherosclerotic vessels a little larger. The vascular connections of coronary artery bypass grafting (CABG), an example, are done with atherosclerotic vessels whose size is on the borderline of those requiring microsurgery, yet the surgical connections have remained open.

Small-artery surgery has found its principal neurosurgical application as EC-IC (first performed in 1967), in which an arterial anastomosis (connecting one vessel to another) is employed, expecting that it will reduce the risk of stroke in selected patients with significant atherosclerotic narrowing (stenosis) of a surgically inaccessible artery to the brain.

For a number of years prior to the introduction of EC-IC, certain patients with diminished circulation to the brain have been subjected to carotid endarterectomy (surgical reconstruction of an accessible artery in their necks). This diminished circulation is usually manifested by brief episodes of weakness, dizziness, and confusion that clear completely within twenty-four hours and are known as TIAs (transient ischemic [deficiency of blood] attacks). TIAs deserve attention because 50 percent of patients with stroke have had one or more premonitory TIA attacks; furthermore, the annual risk of stroke with untreated TIAs is about 10 percent (Winslow, 1988). Thus, successful treatment of the cause of TIAs might prevent stroke. In cases where the TIA is due to an atherosclerotic narrowing of the carotid artery (a main artery which courses up through the neck), carotid endarterectomy (cleaning out the artery) has helped (see below).

When the narrowed artery lies deeper within the head than the carotid, the surgeon may perform an EC-IC bypass. He takes an artery from the temple (superficial temporal artery) and connects it (anastomoses it) to an artery inside the skull (middle cerebral) beyond the point of narrowing. We have here, once more, a reasonable-sounding plan.

Pleased with the technique, neurosurgeons have used EC-IC for indications other than TIAs: recent strokes, small strokes, or other evidence of decreased cerebral circulation. Early in their experience with it, they found that EC-IC didn't work for the emergency treatment of an acute stroke, but they reported many good results among other cases. Patients had fewer TIAs, they felt stronger, went back to work, etc.; investigators even found some evidence that brain circulation was improved. But the clinical end point is critical: Does the operation prevent strokes and lengthen life?

After surgeons had used this inadequately tested operation for ten years, medical scientists in 1977 finally started a multicenter, randomized clinical test. Did the operation decrease the rate of stroke and stroke-related deaths (EC/IC Bypass, 1985)? The test showed that EC-IC failed. Though the bypass remained open in 96 percent of cases—an impressive achievement in itself—the operation didn't seem to help. Nonfatal and fatal strokes occurred both more frequently and earlier in the patients operated upon.

Surgical clinical tests will always be more difficult to conduct than medical clinical tests, but most observers considered this particular test a model—just the kind of trial needed to evaluate unproved therapy. Nonetheless, as has always been the case when a randomized clinical test challenges a popular treatment, rebuttals quickly appeared (Relman, 1987). Its defect, the critics said, was the exclusion of cases. Many patients at the participating institutions had undergone bypass surgery outside the trial, so their possible effect on the results remains unknown. In counterargument, defenders of the trial quoted Francis Bacon: "For what a man had rather were true, he more readily believes" (Barnett et al., 1987).

The clinical trial furnishes strong evidence against the operation. It can't be much good if evidence for its merit is so hard to salvage from the completed clinical test, but some neurosurgeons still believe in it. If EC-IC is offered to you, say no. Warning: In this country, we have an oversupply of neurosurgeons who must keep busy to survive; the very highest medical malpractice insurance rates burden them with an enormous overhead; some of them may try to cling to any income source.

Alternative treatments address the features of health and behavior that lead to stroke—the risk factors (Grotta, 1987). High blood pressure stands first, so have your high blood pressure remedied. Stop smoking, drink less, cut out caffeine, start exercising, eat a low-fat diet, live the modern, healthy life. Heart disease, diabetes, migraine, the use of oral contraceptives, and advanced age are all risk factors. Age you can't avoid, but you may find some encouragement in knowing that stroke's incidence has declined nearly 50 percent during the past thirty years, much of the decline among elderly persons.

A prophylactic treatment, rather than elimination of a risk factor, aspirin, taken regularly after TIAs, reduces the incidence of stroke. And if the cause of your symptoms is atherosclerosis of the carotid artery, carotid endarterectomy may help.

CAROTID ENDARTERECTOMY

When atherosclerosis has narrowed the carotid artery, this operation may reduce the risk of stroke. It has been used in patients with TIAs, in those who have had a stroke, in those with a stroke in "evolution," or in those who with no symptoms are at high risk for stroke (Winslow, 1988b). A 500 percent increase in this operation's use since 1971, with now about 100,000 a year, attests to its popularity, yet there is still a lack of data on its efficacy. A controlled study carried out between 1962 and 1968 concluded that death or stroke associated with the operation negated any long-term protection (Grotta, 1987). The risk of major complications (10 percent) or death (3 percent) severely limits its value. The combined operation—coronary artery bypass and carotid endarterectomy—has increased this operation's risk.

A committee of the American Neurological Association concluded that in patients with TIAs, "carotid endarterectomy may be of value, provided the procedures are performed with a very low surgical complication rate."

But the complication and mortality risk, particularly in older patients, seems too high in general for prophylactic surgery such as this.

A study by UCLA and the Rand corporation on the appropriateness of carotid endarterectomy, reported recently (Winslow, 1988b), casts still another cloud over this operation. The investigation asked a panel of nationally known experts to rate the appropriateness of 864 possible reasons for doing the operation. Using this rating system they then determined—in a random sample of 1,302 Medicare patients in three geographic areas who had the operation in 1981—whether or not surgery was justified. Thirty-five percent had the operation for appropriate reasons, 32 percent for equivocal reasons, and 32 percent for inappropriate reasons. Most of the inappropriate operations were done on arteries with minimal stenosis, on patients with high surgical risk, or on arteries on the wrong side in view of the symptoms. Compared with EC-ICs, which are perhaps never done for good reasons, carotid endarterectomy is of some use. But with only one third done for what experts consider appropriate reasons, it represents a shocking overuse of surgery nonetheless.

If your doctor has recommended this operation, be sure to get a second opinion, and if you can, find out what the complication rate is in your hospital. Understand what you are getting into. If you have any doubt, hold off, go for the same alternatives listed for EC-IC.

Is there anything else? Yes, unfortunately. Surgeons in Italy, England, China, and Japan, we are told, have been taking a pad of fat (the omentum) from the belly and stitching it on to the exposed brain in order to improve circulation (Help for Stroke, 1987). As you might expect, they have reported good results. Says Mark Ravitch, prominent American surgeon: "The first report of any new operation is rarely unfavorable." More than your good sense will protect you from this operation because surgeons in the United States have been reluctant to take it up—so far.

VARICOSE VEINS

On her fiftieth birthday Carol R. decided to have something done about her veins. She hated wearing pants and support hose all the time. Her figure was still trim, and her legs would be shapely—if it weren't for the damn veins.

The surgeon she consulted spent a lot of time fussing around, examining her legs: She had to lie down, stand up with tight rubber tubes around her legs in various locations. Finally he spoke: "Both the large and the small saphenous veins are incompetent on the right, and the large saphenous on the left." With his index finger he traced the course of these veins along the insides of her legs from the thigh down to the ankle, and on the back of her right calf. "But the deep veins seem to be okay. You can wear support hose okay, can't you?"

"Oh, sure," said Carol, "they make my legs feel better, but I'm sick of wearing them all the time, and they're so ugly."

"The skin on the middle side of your ankle here," he touched her right ankle just above the ankle bone, "is darker than the rest. Do you know how long it's been like that?"

Carol rubbed the spot, brownish, slightly blue or pink around the edges. "It itches. I don't know, maybe a year."

"Something like that could . . . ah, flare up, cause more trouble. It's a good reason for having the veins removed."

"I'd like to get rid of them all right, but how about injections?" Needles! Who wants needles? "Maybe you don't believe in shots," she said. Maybe she didn't believe in them either, but she pushed on: "My neighbor, Bernice, says she had injections, and they helped a lot."

"No, you have too many varicose veins, and some of them are too big. Of course, we might have to do some injections to clean up what's left after the surgery."

"Well, I guess I could ask Billy . . . but he'd say to do what I think is best." She paused, "So, okay, I guess. But what if I need the veins later for my heart?" She brightened up. "I've heard about that. My cousin, Dan, I guess you don't know him, who is over sixty now, had a bypass, and his wife told me they used veins from his legs."

"Yeah, they probably did," said the surgeon, "but your veins are pretty badly shot to be of much use. Instead they can use small arteries from the chest for a bypass. Eventually they may have good artificial blood vessels, or bypasses may no longer be needed. In any case, your heart seems to be perfectly okay now. You'll probably never need a bypass."

Carol's varicose veins were "ligated and stripped" under general anesthesia. When she awoke she found both her legs wrapped in thick bandages from her toes to her hips, but despite this handicap the stern nurses rousted her out of bed to walk in the hall as soon as she was fully conscious. When the bandages were finally removed, she counted ten short incisions on her right leg and six on her left. Her legs remained black and blue for a couple of weeks, and the scars never completely disappeared, but except for a couple of small veins on the back of her right calf, which the surgeon injected three weeks after surgery, the ugly veins had disappeared. By six months the discolored spot on her right ankle had almost faded away; itching had ceased long before that.

Even if you have varicose veins, you may avoid surgery if you want to. Most victims can. In surgery's favor, however, is its relative safety and effectiveness. If you hate those tortuous, blue destroyers of surface beauty, you might as well go ahead (unless you are pregnant).

Physicians have been treating varicose veins for more than a couple of millennia (Flye, 1986). Hippocrates, the famous Greek physician, described them 2,500 years ago. He did not understand the circulation of the blood (Harvey discovered that in 1628, over 2,000 years later), but he could see that something was wrong. Common now and throughout history, varicosities—legs are their usual location—are an obvious abnormality. Twenty million people in the United States have them, and about 50,000 submit to surgery each year.

Distended, convoluted veins are found in many parts of the body; for example, hemorrhoids (see next chapter) may be a type of varicose vein. Varicose veins occur most often in the two major superficial veins of the legs, just beneath the skin: The greater saphenous, which runs up the inner side of the leg from the middle side of the ankle to the upper thigh, and the lesser saphenous, which courses up the calf from the ankle to the back of the knee. Although varicose veins may appear all over the surface of the legs, their source vein is either the greater or lesser saphenous vein.

The trouble begins as a valve failure in these veins. Normal venous valves permit the blood to flow only toward the heart, and muscle action, as in walking, pushes the blood along. When the valves fail, blood backs up, the veins distend, sometimes the blood even flows the wrong way. If the deep veins located within the muscles, into which the backed-up blood flows, are sound, they will then carry the entire load. The superficial, varicose veins are then no longer needed, and they may actually be a handicap. Their ruined valves will never recover.

Exclusively a disease of humans, varicose veins are blamed on our upright posture, but heredity plays a big part. Furthermore, a standing occupation may provoke the trouble, and pregnancy certainly does. About one fifth of pregnant women develop varicose veins, which usually vanish after delivery. Some physician theorists say that constipation may bring on varicose veins, and everyone agrees that, as with so many of our afflictions, they are often a disease of aging—a bit of the final wreck.

They have been treated with puncture, avulsion (detachment), excision, cautery, ligation (tying off), resection (removal) injection, or stripping; perhaps, too, with unctions, ointments, and spells, but here the record fails us. Too aggressively treated? If you want to get rid of the pesky things, you may have to root them out aggressively, one by one.

At the charity hospital where I trained, as their first operation, surgical interns were permitted to tie off the greater saphenous vein where it joins a deeper vein in the upper thigh—an operation we called ligation. The varicosities, now disconnected from the main venous system, were expected to shrink and finally disappear or surrender to later injections. This was performed on outpatients under local anesthesia.

One afternoon an elderly man, who had hobbled painfully one block from the hospital to the streetcar stop following such an operation, tried to climb the steps of the trolley's rear platform. He stretched himself a little too far, and the tied-off stump of his greater saphenous vein burst. To the horror of fellow passengers, a great gush of blood poured onto the platform, cascading through its grille floor to the street. The large vein that runs from the thigh, where the stump had blown, to the heart has no valves to impede a disastrous backflow.

The man collapsed, but he did survive—doubtless saved by the resulting drop in central venous pressure and by the pressure on the wound applied by one adroit witness. (In the vicinity of a hospital, where employees go to and fro on the streets, you may be lucky enough to encounter someone truly capable of first aid.)

By the way, my colleague Jim, who had done the operation, changed specialties after finishing his surgical internship. He then trained to become a psychiatrist.

Later our hospital began admitting patients for varicose vein surgery, and its surgeons switched to the more painstaking modern operation called ligation and stripping—an operation your surgeon will doubtless use. Depending upon where the varicosities are located, the greater saphenous vein, the lesser saphenous vein, or both are ligated. Then using flexible probes passed through the veins and multiple small incisions, the varicose veins are actually torn (stripped) out.

If you intend to have such an operation mainly to improve appearance, you can expect that the operation will rid you of the unsightly veins, but you'll have small scars, as many as ten or so per leg, not easy to hide under sheer stockings. If you had skin changes due to the veins, they will disappear, but slowly. As in the case of Carol R., a skin thinning and discoloration on the inside just above the ankle is one compelling indication for surgery, as is skin weeping or an ulcer in the same area—advanced stages of the disease. Other noncosmetic indications for the operation are large varicosities that may be injured and severe symptoms such as aching, heaviness, and leg cramps. Pregnancy is a contraindication to surgery, and atherosclerosis with diminished blood supply may be, though varicose veins and atherosclerosis are unrelated diseases. Veins, by the way, don't acquire atherosclerosis, as do arteries, unless they are transplanted to the arterial system—the fate of the greater saphenous vein when used as the bypass channel in the coronary bypass operation.

Atherosclerosis of the venous bypass graft, one of the late complications of coronary bypass, causes dissatisfaction with venous grafts. Nonetheless, the possible need of a vein graft for CABG has reduced the incidence of varicose vein surgery. If this is what is keeping you from having such surgery, forget it. Small arteries serve better than a vein in CABG; furthermore, if you ever do need a CABG something will probably have come along to replace the vein—or to replace the CABG. It's happening already.

In contrast to heart surgery, varicose-vein surgery remains static. Surgeons have been using ligation and stripping for forty years or more, with good results. The Mayo Clinic, for example, reports satisfactory results in 94 percent of their patients after five years and in 85 percent after ten years.

The operation has never been subjected to the prospective, random, clinical testing I have been harping about. Results in various grades of the disease have never been carefully compared with the results of alternative treatments or with no treatment. We don't know as much as we'd like to know, but for most cases we know about as much as we need to know. When done for appearance's sake, the operation removes the unsightly veins more durably than do injections. For advanced disease, as in a leg with ulcers, there is no effective alternative to surgery.

When the main indication is cosmetic, however, and the veins are small, injections provide a satisfactory alternative. An irritating solution is injected into the collapsed varicose vein, causing it to clot, become obstructed, and finally turn into a fibrous cord. Unfortunately, good results don't last as long as results following surgery. In one series of 284 patients, 89 percent had good results after three months, but only 68 percent had good results after three to four years. You may have to go back for more injections.

Other alternatives are elastic bandages or support hose. Some medical-supply companies will fashion hose to fit your leg precisely. Exercise seems to help too—most effectively as a preventive. And, as I said at the beginning, the majority of varicose veins do not have to be treated. If you have no symptoms, no skin changes, and no longing for youthful, surface beauty, hide them beneath trousers or support hose and carry on.

5

Piles

If your doctor has recommended a hemorrhoidectomy, he has assigned you to a small minority. Piles are very common, but few victims require surgery. Some authorities say half the people of the United States over the age of fifty have hemorrhoids; others push the proportion higher—as much as 70 percent of those over age forty. An old Chinese proverb states, "Nine out of every ten men have piles." The disease *is* common. Despite its commonness, however, fewer patients are being subjected to hemorrhoidectomy: 128,000 in 1984, 109,000 in 1986. The operation is faulty, and alternative treatments suffice.

A.J., a forty-three-year-old accountant, felt a burning when his bowels moved, particularly if they were loose. Most of the time, though, he was constipated, and when he strained to defecate, a lump of something would protrude from his anus. When he touched this with an exploring finger, he became frightened. Cancer? He delayed, didn't go to the doctor until he noticed blood on the toilet paper and a spot on his underwear.

After examining A.J.'s rectum and colon with special instruments, the doctor had no trouble making up *his* mind: piles, not cancer. A.J. took the option the doctor offered and checked into the hospital to have the piles removed surgically. He lay there, restless under spinal anesthesia, jackknifed on an operating table with his rear end uppermost and exposed under a brilliant light, while the surgeon worked on him.

After the operation they didn't let him leave the hospital until he had a bowel movement. Now, he told his wife, he knew what it must feel like to bear a child. (The wife smiled sardonically.) The doctor had him back every few days to stretch the healing anus—necessary to prevent strictures, he said—and for three weeks A.J. took sitz baths after every bowel movement. It still hurt to move his bowels, but less in time. More annoyance: When his bowels were a little loose, he tended to soil his underwear. This he controlled by diet, by exercising his anal sphincter muscle, and by spending less time seated. Two years after the operation, he received a follow-up letter from his surgeon asking him to return for a checkup, but A.J. didn't return.

Surgeons have extirpated piles in a vast number of ways, and, dissatisfied with their handiwork, they have also devised a variety of clever nonsurgical treatments—based sometimes on unprecedented theories of the disease's origin. The many kinds of operations advocated may mean either that none of them are much good or that anything works—after a fashion. The odd theories of causation may mean that not enough is really known about this ancient disease. In any case, delay before you agree to an operation for piles. Choose a conservative treatment first.

HISTORY

Surgeons, who were once merely humble technicians or barbers doing surgery on the side, owe their ascent to a respectable social status to a royal hemorrhoidal intervention. In seventeenth century France, the surgeon Felix successfully treated Louis XIV's anal fistula (a complication of hemorrhoids), and the king promptly made Felix and his successor, George Mareschal, royal surgeons (Garrison, 1929). The Paris Faculty, nonsurgeons to a man, objected, but the surgeons held fast.

Before and since that French episode, surgeons have thought a lot about this indelicate disease and its complications. Hippocrates in the fifth century B.C., known to this day for the physician's ethical code, the Hippocratic Oath, had learned to treat anal fistula by passing a ligature through the fistula and allowing it to work its way through the tissue, joining the fistula to the anus (Zimmerman and Veith, 1961)—a technique still popular and successful today. Later, in ancient Salerno, physicians used other methods to treat hemorrhoids, which have not endured as well. With a background of Greek, Roman, and Arabic teachings, they passed on this recommendation: "For hemorrhoids, take some of the little worms which are found under stones, the kind that are rough on the outside with a great many feet but roll up into a ball when you disturb them. Boil them in linseed oil and apply the oil to the place" (Graham, 1939). Worms found under rocks, boiling oil, cutting, excising, sewing, binding, it seems that everything has been tried, but surgeons still search. They have failed to find and commit themselves to one best way.

CAUSE

Moreover, they have failed to agree on the cause and the nature of the disease. It's a disease of man, that's clear, a disease of upright, sedentary, broad-bottomed, constipated man. As early as 1769, Giovanni Morgagni, an Italian pathologist, attributed hemorrhoids to increased pressure from the upright posture—a presumed cause of varicose veins as well, as we learned in the last chapter (Thomson, 1975). Hemorrhoids look like varicose veins, and the dogma accepted by most modern proctologists is that hemorrhoids are rectal-vein varicosities. But some object and claim that they are really normal "cushions" that have been displaced, or that they are due not to increased pressure at all but to a narrowing of the rectum (Hancock and Smith, 1975), while others claim that infection is the principal cause. Heredity seems to play a part too, but it's hard to be sure when so many people in all hereditary lines have the disease.

All agree that child-bearing brings them on. "Women during the state of pregnancy, and just after the menses have finally left them, are peculiarly subject to the piles," said William Heberden, an English physician, of the eighteenth century. Heart failure or cirrhosis of the liver may cause them, because pressure on the veins is increased by these conditions, and they are frequently provoked by diarrhea or constipation—by straining.

They *are* a disease of constipated, worried man, so mental attitude plays a part, too. Psychiatrists, in their windy ways, say that because of the rich symbolism associated with feces and all that, and because the function of the anus is partially under voluntary control, constipation may be psychological (Engel, 1975). Perhaps, therefore, you could cure your hemorrhoids by renovating your psychological furnishings or by just learning to relax.

INDICATIONS FOR SURGERY

Or you might not have to bother at all. Most hemorrhoids cause no symptoms and don't predispose to any further trouble, other than to an aggravation of themselves. (This aggravation may be prevented by the habits and diet I will describe in "Alternatives to Surgery.") When aggravation does occur, the common symptoms are bleeding, itching, pain, soiling, and protrusion of the hemorrhoid through the anus.

Internal hemorrhoids form inside and are covered with the mucosa, the lining of the bowel. If large, they may show themselves by protruding through the anus. External hemorrhoids are outside from the start; they form external to the anal margin, but close to it, and are covered with skin. Mixed hemorrhoids show features of both external and internal hemorrhoids (Bubrick and Benjamin, 1985).

Along with this external-internal classification, hemorrhoids may be categorized according to severity. First degree: protrude minimally, symptoms chiefly painless bleeding. Second degree: protrude through the anus during straining, but go back up spontaneously when straining stops. Third degree: protrude with less effort and have to be pushed back with the fingers. Fourth degree: protrude all the time, can't be pushed back in.

If your doctor has recommended surgery, the treatment he or his referral surgeon proposes will likely depend upon the degree: less radical therapy for degrees one or two, hemorrhoidectomy for degree three or four. But even if your hemorrhoids are large, consider delay. Ask if you couldn't try nonoperative measures first. If your doctor has examined your rectum and colon above the site of the hemorrhoids (proctoscopy, colonoscopy), as he should, and you have no other disease higher up, such as cancer, there's no hurry. The operation hurts, convalescence drags on. With careful cleansing, rest, and diet, you may recover without surgery. Commonly, I believe, the improvement that follows surgery results from the postoperative care (sitz baths, rest, etc.) as much as from the operation itself. That kind of care will promote healing despite the operation.

THE OPERATION—HEMORRHOIDECTOMY

During a hemorrhoidectomy the surgeon excises the hemorrhoids, usually in three locations around the circumference of the anus; then he sews up the wounds (Corman, 1988). Simple enough, but trouble comes from the contamination and the traffic. You can't rid the anus of its germs, and you can't rest the operative site for long. Stool accumulates and must find its way out. Healing is like trying to grow grass in the playground. The wounds are contaminated from the start and always sensitive. The first bowel movement postop? Like having "a barbed wire pulled through the rectum," said an articulate victim.

Healing may be slow and irregular. In order to prevent stricture and the dreaded late complication of stenosis (a narrowed anus), the surgeon may feel obliged to dilate the healing anus with his finger. I've seen an anus not subjected to dilation following hemorrhoidectomy that scarred down to the diameter of a lead pencil. Stools that narrow are a great bother.

To manage the problems of an infected wound, some surgeons have intentionally left the wounds partially open, to heal secondarily. More common these days is a "closed" operation in which the wounds are sewn up, but in either case, infection and slow healing are bugbears. Damage to the sphincter muscle resulting in incontinence, tender scars, and hemorrhoid recurrence are other late complications.

RESULTS

Nonetheless, good results following surgery are usually reported by surgeons with experience: 90 percent patient satisfaction, only 0.5 percent having lasting incontinence, 7 percent needing further treatment, and so forth (McConnell and Khubchandani, 1983). Here, as with so many popular operations, there have never been any random, controlled, clinical tests comparing results of surgery with nonoperative treatment. Lacking such tests, the operation is on uncertain clinical grounds; its indications equivocal.

Examination of the operative specimen by a pathologist may provide a convenient way to monitor some operations, but not hemorrhoidectomy. If the surgeon removes a gallbladder, the pathologist would expect it to show stones or at least *some* pathology. With hemorrhoids, however, what can he say? All he has to examine are a few beat-up veins. Did the piles really have to be removed? Can't tell.

OTHER OPERATIONS

Less radical operations than hemorrhoidectomy have turned up all over the place as office procedures—often first in England, because there they have long waiting lists for elective hospital surgery. The new techniques are quicker, cheaper, less painful; maybe they are as good, at least for first- and second-degree piles. Or maybe they aren't needed at all—hard to tell. If your doctor has recommended one of them, and you want to have something done, you will probably find one of them easier to endure than a hemorrhoidectomy.

Injection: To inject a hemorrhoid, the surgeon inserts a tube (a proctoscope) into the rectum, locates the hemorrhoid, and shoots a sclerosing solution (an irritating mixture of quinine and urea hydrochloride) into it with a syringe and needle. The blood in the hemorrhoid clots, the hemorrhoid itself wastes away, the resulting raw area heals, and only a scar remains. St. Marks hospital in London, a famous place for colon and rectal diseases, reports that they use injection for 75 percent of their cases (Thompson, 1977).

Rubber-band ligation: After locating the hemorrhoid through a proctoscope, the operator grabs the hemorrhoid with a forceps and stretches it out a little. Then he slips a gun, on which special, small, strong rubber bands have been mounted, over both the forceps and the hemorrhoid and ejects a rubber band from the gun to surround the base of the hemorrhoid tightly, strangulating it. When, later, the dead hemorrhoid drops off, the rubber band drops off with it. If you have several hemorrhoids, you may need more than one visit. Simple technique. But any operation has its complications, and one of the complications of this operation has been grim. Four deaths have been reported due to sepsis following rubber-band ligation (Bubrick and Benjamin, 1985).

A random clinical test has been used to compare injection of a sclerosing solution with rubber-band ligation. Rubber bands won out, and there were no serious complications in either group.

The most surprising of the new, less-radical techniques has been anal dilatation (Lord, 1968). Under general anesthesia, the canal is simply dilated—to the extent of all four fingers of both hands. Whew! You could deliver a small baby through that opening. After this effort the surgeon stops; he ignores the hemorrhoids. But the hemorrhoids shrink anyway, and the canal quickly recovers its normal size and function—they say. English proctologists have publicized the method, but it has not caught on in this country largely because of concern about sphincter injury and postoperative incontinence. By the way, since anal dilatation—though not quite as ample as this English dilatation—is carried out as part of most hemorrhoidectomies, could dilatation itself be the important part of the operation, not the cutting and stitching?

Surgeons are by nature mechanics and apt to take up with new machines. They have applied several, relatively new, destructive devices to the hemorrhoid. For instance, your surgeon might subject your hemorrhoids to such physical agents as freezing (cryosurgery), infrared coagulation (heat), and most recently various kinds of laser beams. These methods neatly dispatch the hemorrhoid, but they are probably not decisively better at it than injection or the rubber-band technique—just more expensive.

Occasionally for a thrombosed (blood-clotted) hemorrhoid, a painful complication, another minor operation may help you. If your doctor wants to lance your thrombosed hemorrhoid or excise it under local anesthesia, let him. When a clot forms in an external pile, the pile swells and becomes acutely painful. If lanced under local anesthesia, the clot pops out, and the pressure is relieved. You may, however, not need even this minor surgery. Try hot sitz baths. For many hemorrhoid troubles, alternatives to surgery work.

ALTERNATIVES TO SURGERY

For acute problems, such as a thrombosed hemorrhoid, the measures used to speed healing following hemorrhoidectomy may help. Bed rest reduces the venous pressure due to upright posture—itself a possible cause of hemorrhoids—and sitz baths (sitting in a tub of hot water) cleans and soothes the ailment.

For any type of hemorrhoids bowel control is essential. After surgery, your surgeon may prescribe mineral oil to smooth the passage, but for the long haul and to avoid the need for surgery in the first place, a diet with bran and fiber to soften and increase the bulk of your stools and thereby prevent constipation will help. Also, cut down on use of milk products. If bowels move easily, hemorrhoids tend to heal themselves. Sometimes bulk laxatives such as psyllium seed products, as found in Metamucil, will help. Drink a lot of water; the fiber will absorb it and become soft.

Commercial ointments may relieve the itching and irritation, but to speed healing and for long-term control, keep the area clean. Don't be afraid to use soap and water; you may have to become well enough acquainted with your own anatomy so that you can thoroughly wash the piles and push them back inside. Water is a gentler and more effective cleanser than toilet paper. If you have had a flare-up, try to bathe the area with soap and water after every bowel movement—take a shower or use a bidet (if you can find one). No wound, even a minor one, heals well in a contaminated environment, and without scrupulous cleansing, no surface area is more contaminated than the anus—unless it's the mouth.

6

Prostatectomy

Had your doctor's recommendation for prostate surgery come at the turn of the century, he might have recommended castration, and that radical extirpation of otherwise healthy but allied organs might actually have helped, for the prostate *is* sensitive to male hormones. It grows with their administration, shrinks with their lack. Castration may still be used occasionally for prostate cancer, but not today for the most common prostate affliction (BPH—benign prostatic hypertrophy). If it's BPH, the doctor will advocate excising part or all of the gland itself (prostatectomy)—by one route or another.

We don't find much about the prostate in early medical writings, perhaps because its diseases are diseases of old men, and there weren't that many old men about, or it may have escaped attention because the gland lies deep in the pelvis, not easily noticed until it blocks the bladder's output—a hidden walnut fed by age and male hormones to outgrow its narrow space. Located in front of the rectum and at the outlet of the bladder, it can enlarge (hypertrophy, the medical term) to the size of an orange. That much growth in that small space impedes or even stops the flow of urine.

FUNCTION AND MALFUNCTION

Like testicles and penis, the prostate, a genital organ, is found only in males. It consists of glandular and fibrous tissue enclosed in a connective tissue capsule. Within the center of the gland the spermatic duct, which carries sperm from the testicles, joins the urethra, a tube which leads from the bladder to the end of the penis. Thus the urethra will carry at times urine, sperm, or prostatic secretion in various mixtures. The prostate secretion is the semen, a thick whitish fluid with which the sperm is mixed before ejaculation. As in any organ, prostatic cells divide and reproduce to replace worn-out tissue, but sometimes this cell-replacement process becomes too active and disordered, producing a benign tumor (BPH— benign prostatic hypertrophy), or cancer (adenocarcinoma).

PAST AND PRESENT

Shortly after the turn of the century, an English surgeon and an East Coast urologist began excising the prostate, and urologists have been at it ever since. The East Coast urologist, by the way, was Hugh Young who, among his other accomplishments, successfully removed Diamond Jim Brady's bladder stone in 1912 with a punch instrument he had developed and used to take out parts of the prostate (Meade, 1968; Brown, 1986). Thereupon in 1915 the grateful and fabulously wealthy Diamond Jim endowed a new urological institute for Johns Hopkins Medical School, the James Buchanan Brady Urological Institute—subsequently the source of much distinguished urological work.

Prostatectomy, as with dental-plaque-awareness and toupee wearers, is increasing (U.S. Department of Health and Human Services, 1986). At over 300,000 a year, it is now one of the most common operations in the U.S. About 60 percent of sixty-year-old men have some prostate trouble; by age eighty-five, 95 percent of them have complaints. So, there's bound to be plenty of interest; and old men, when they have power over the economics of medical investigation (as they do in Congress), will advocate "further investigation." Should these old men lose power, somewhat younger men, with similar enduring concerns for their male organs, prevail.

Surprising, then, that we know so little about the gland and its diseases. Nevertheless, as shown by the experience of a couple of our political leaders, treatment has improved. Thomas Jefferson, our third President, suffered from complications of a prostate that blocked his urine flow

("Prostate," 1987) and as a consequence he experienced uremia (backing up of blood chemicals ordinarily secreted in the urine). Hearing of his trouble, the Marquis de LaFayette shipped him an early French version of the urethral catheter, which might have emptied Jefferson's obstructed bladder. But it arrived too late, and Jefferson died of prostate trouble and the failure of slow communication.

Benjamin Franklin, another founding father, also suffered prostate trouble. We are told that he eased the discomfort caused to his distended bladder by bouncing travel by designing a specially sprung carriage for the rough rides on cobbled Philadelphia streets.

Ronald Reagan, our fortieth president, has had two prostatic operations, one in 1967 when he was fifty-six and the second in 1986 when he was seventy-five. The modern operation, still the only effective treatment for his disease, BPH, hardly slowed him up.

BPH—BENIGN PROSTATIC HYPERTROPHY

BPH, a noncancerous prostatic overgrowth, begins after age forty. It reaches its highest frequency between sixty and seventy, peaking in blacks about five years earlier (Grayhack, 1976). Most men over sixty have some prostatic enlargement, and many have a few symptoms. If they do, long periods of remission or temporary standstill may allow them to avoid surgery, but once it starts to grow, the prostate tends to keep on growing. This enlargement may finally require a prostatectomy. In fact, some urologists have estimated that a fifty-year-old man has a 20 to 25 percent chance of requiring a prostatectomy during his lifetime (Walsh, 1986). Urologists haven't mustered that many candidates for surgery yet, but they do a big business.

CAUSE

Search for a cause goes on. Because young males and eunuchs of any age don't incur BPH, we know that aging and the presence of testes are required. There are no clear risk factors, such as tobacco for lung cancer and high blood pressure for stroke. Risk of BPH is unrelated to social class, marital status, celibacy (Catholic priests get it too), "sexual drive," smoking, or anything else. Though some authorities believe that BPH may be a precursor to cancer of the prostate, most say that it isn't.

NATURAL HISTORY

Fifteen to twenty years may pass from the inception of BPH to the onset of symptoms—caused, finally, by urine outflow obstruction or by irritation of the bladder or urethra. Frequency, urgency, and a dribbling incontinence may then embarrass the subject. The stream narrows and loses its normal trajectory; the victim may have to strain to start what turns out to be no more than an interrupted flow; even worse, he may suddenly not be able to pass anything at all (acute retention).

Chronic infection and the backup caused by obstruction can ruin the kidneys, and because of this, the disease causes significant worldwide mortality. Men in many backward regions may succumb to kidney failure as Thomas Jefferson did 160 years ago. You should not ignore evidence of this disease. Nonetheless, if your symptoms are only mild and nonprogressive, you may avoid surgery. Many men untreated will have no change in their symptoms for years. When *is* surgery indicated?

INDICATIONS

If infection, severe bleeding, or obstruction that threatens kidney function appears, you need a prostatectomy. A sudden complete obstruction will also, in most cases, require prostatectomy. On the other hand, if your only manifestation of the disease is the need to get up a couple of times during the night, you may not need surgery. Maybe you'll never need it.

A textbook of urology lists as one of its indications for surgery: "Outflow obstructive symptoms that are of sufficient concern to the patient to cause him to desire treatment (Walsh, 1986)." Vague indeed. This opens the door to a lot of surgery that we could get along without. If your symptoms are only mild, urologists really don't know when the operation is indicated, so they leave it up to you. Should your urologist present the matter of surgery to you this way, there is obviously no hurry. Like many operations we are considering, prostatectomy for mild BPH has not been subjected to random, controlled tests comparing it with nonoperative management.

As an alternative to such tests, and the best they could do without them, J. E. Wennberg and his associates have undertaken, as an example of what is known as "patient-outcome" research, a prostatectomy assessment project (Barry et al., 1988; Fowler et al., 1988; Wennberg et al., 1988). They examined the available data and found a striking geographical variation in the incidence of prostatectomy, denoting that supposed experts disagree on how to treat an individual patient. In some places the experts operate; in other places, for the same symptoms they don't. Factors such as the urologist's specialty training, clinical experience, and personal characteristics; the patient's personal characteristics; and the economics of the area may influence the decision to operate more than does evidence of clinical need.

Wennberg and his associates state: "The clinical sources of unwanted variations in prostatectomy rates appear to be due to a lack of information concerning the risks and benefits of the procedure, an inappropriate belief that the operation prolongs life, and a failure to base decisions on patient preferences for outcomes." Regarding patient preference they further state: "When operations that carry risks are undertaken primarily to improve the quality of life, the threshold should appropriately vary from patient to patient, according to the strength of their feelings about their symptoms and their attitudes toward risk" (Barry, 1988).

You as a patient must be sure that you understand your options. For all but chronic, severe obstruction, watchful waiting may be best.

THE OPERATION

In the language of urologists the operation is either "open" or "closed." They perform an "open" operation through a skin incision, and a "closed" operation through a long, narrow tube, in this case a resectoscope, which is passed up the penis.

Most urologists have used a closed operation, though a recent report, with surprising results suggesting that it is less effective and perhaps more risky than an open operation, may change this (Roos et al., 1989). In a transurethral (meaning across or through the urethra) resection of the prostate (TURP), done under spinal or general anesthesia, the operator introduces the resectoscope through the penis, and while peering into a fiberoptic view system, which has been improved enormously since the days of Hugh Young and Diamond Jim Brady, he uses electrical currents and special instruments to scoop the gland out piecemeal.

P.N., a seventy-two-year-old lawyer, had been getting up two or three times at night to urinate. After a couple of years of this, he suddenly passed a gush of bright red blood. When his doctor had finished examining him and x-raying his kidneys, he said, "Your kidneys are fine, but your prostate has grown too large. I think you ought to have it out before it gets any bigger." The urologist at a prominent Midwest clinic, to which P.N. had journeyed for a second opinion, agreed, and P.N. had a TURP for his BPH.

A year later, two days before Christmas, while visiting his children, P.N. noticed blood in his urine again, and he had great difficulty urinating. The urologist he saw then removed a blood clot from the bladder and used an instrument to open up a stricture (narrowing) that had formed at the previous site of the prostate. Back home P.N. still had difficulty urinating; following an unskilled catheterization at a local emergency room, he developed chills, fever, and a bloodstream infection. Antibiotics caused a drug reaction with shock and diarrhea. More, but different antibiotics, didn't immediately subdue the infection, but a third antibiotic finally did.

Eighteen months postoperatively, he bled once again. Could I have cancer? he asked himself. No, said the urologist, just an unhealed spot at the outlet of the bladder, at the site of the TURP; it's healing slowly. Using the same operating cystoscope he might use for a TURP, the urologist then excised this slowly healing area to give the wound a fresh start. P.N. left the hospital in three days but came back bleeding once more. He was given a new antibiotic and had another drug reaction, from which he recovered when, finally, all the antibiotics were stopped.

Now, eight months after this last episode, he only bleeds a little off and on, but he still has to get up a couple of times at night to urinate (as he did before surgery). He has an inguinal hernia which he attributes to all the straining he has had to do in order to pee. Soon, at the same clinic where he had the TURP, he will have the hernia repaired. Is he impotent? Well, yes, sort of, he says, but he doesn't think the TURP had anything to do with *that*. When asked if he is pleased to have had the TURP, he says, "Yes, of course." He thinks the operation was required.

A TURP doesn't necessarily cause impotence. In one series of 100 men who were potent preoperatively, only fourteen were impotent postoperatively (*Prevention*, 1980). In another, however, 46 percent felt that the procedure had a deleterious effect on their potency (Grayhack, 1976). Investigators who look into this matter point out, in support of P.N.'s feeling about his own case, that psychological issues and the natural consequences of aging may have as much to do with impotence as operative damage. While the operation may not cause impotence, it does cause sterility, because the ejaculate goes into the bladder rather than out through the penis. The French, who always have a word for such things, call it *le plaisir sec*, the dry pleasure. But I have heard it described as waiting for an explosion that never comes.

In 20 percent of cases urologists use open operations. If the open operation is to be a perineal prostatectomy, they make an incision between the anus and the scrotum (perineal region) and approach the gland from below, removing it entirely. For a suprapubic prostatectomy, they make an incision in the lower abdomen, enter the urinary bladder, and reach the prostate through the floor of the bladder. With a retropubic prostatectomy, they also make a lower abdominal incision, but then reach the prostate by working down in front of the bladder, without entering it.

RESULTS

With the cooperation of twenty-three urologists in the state of Maine, Wennberg and his associates carried out pre- and postoperative interviews with over 300 patients and supplemented this information with a study of current medical literature, with data on specific patients from health insurance programs, and with assessment by a technique of decision analysis. They found that the operation *did* reduce symptoms—in 93 percent of severely symptomatic and 79 percent of moderately symptomatic patients. However, they found an improvement in "quality of life" (general health, mental health, and activity) only for those who had acute retention or who were most symptomatic before surgery.

Short-term complications occurred in 24 percent of patients—a much higher rate than had been expected. Four percent reported persistent incontinence, and 5 percent of those who were potent before surgery were impotent after surgery. Twenty percent needed a reoperation within eight years. Usually surgeons assume that their complication and reoperation rates will be similar to those in published reports from academic centers, but as these studies showed, actual outcome on the firing line of community practice may be significantly less. Academic centers, too, may find that their unreported outcomes fail to reach the figures they manage to accumulate for publication.

Early operation in patients without chronic obstruction does not extend life expectancy. In fact, because of the risk of postoperative death, prostatectomy results in a slight decrease of average life expectancy.

Urologists have believed that TURP is as effective as an open operation with less risk (mortality about 1 percent for open operations and less than

1 percent for TURP), but a new report by Wennberg and his associates on results with over 50,000 patients in Denmark, England, and Canada may change their beliefs (Roos, et al., 1989). Using patient-outcome research and massive amounts of data from several sources, they concluded that TURP was a less effective operation than open surgery because it required a second prostatectomy more frequently. TURP also had a higher long-term mortality—this not a quite convincing observation, however (Greenfield, 1989). This clinical research, based on new ways of analyzing available data, rather than on the preferred but expensive and difficult randomized clinical trial, has shed important new light on BPH treatment.

Prostatectomy for serious obstruction yields a rapid relief of symptoms in approximately 90–98 percent of cases. Will you need a second operation, as did President Reagan? Will you need a third? "When will that happen? Every twenty years?" asked reporter Sam Donaldson of Larry Speakes, the White House spokesman, when Ronald Reagan had his second operation. "I think he's good for forty years this time," replied Speakes ("Prostate," 1987).

ALTERNATIVES

If your symptoms are mild and stable, forbearance offers the best alternative to surgery. Only surgery will eliminate the disease, however. Drugs, vitamins, whatever will not prevent or cure BPH. As I mentioned earlier, castration will prevent it, but even a modest respect for enduring sexuality rules that out.

The catheter life, too, is a bad deal. I remember men waiting for a TURP who were brought in from the rest home to the outpatient clinic twice a day to have their bladders emptied with a catheter—their lives centered on low fluid intake and that essential, twice-a-day mission. Had they decided not to have the TURP that they were waiting for, they could have carried their own catheter—in the hatband, I have been told—and slipped it into their bladder a couple of times a day until infection caught up with them.

PROSTATIC CANCER

If your doctor has recommended surgery for prostatic cancer, it may not be as bad as you think. And there are good alternatives to surgery that you should be aware of. First, something about the disease.

Rare before age fifty and common after sixty, prostatic cancer is the second most common cause of cancer-related deaths in American men, outranked only by lung. Approximately 96,000 new cases are diagnosed each year, and 26,000 deaths are reported annually (Consensus Conference, 1987). Blacks have a higher incidence than whites, and American Indians, Orientals, and Hispanics have a lower incidence (Catalona and Scott, 1986). It is usually discovered by rectal examination, often incidentally, or it may be found incidentally at prostatectomy for BPH; pathologists find it in more than 10 percent of BPH specimens, undiagnosed before the surgery. One fourth of all American males over the age of seventy, who have died from other causes, can be shown to have small cancers of the prostate (Cairns, 1985) as well, and some investigators contend that it can be found microscopically in 35 percent of men past age fifty. Many of these incidentally discovered cancers grow slowly, of course, and do not cause symptoms. In fact, only about one third of prostatic cancers become clinically manifest during a person's lifetime.

CAUSE

Although the root cause of prostate cancer is unknown, heredity apparently plays a part, and hormones control its inception and growth. Eunuchs don't have cancer of the prostate, and castration or female-hormone administration affects the growth of an established cancer. The observation that second generation Japanese men contract it as commonly as other United States natives, while their fathers, brought up in Japan, have a lower incidence implies that exposure to as yet unidentified chemical agents in the environment may be an inciting cause. Possibly an infectious agent, sexually transmitted, plays a part. In any case, the disease is more common in men who have been sexually active and in men who have had venereal disease (Catalona and Scott, 1986).

NATURAL HISTORY

It may remain undetected throughout life, or spread quietly and then first become evident because of symptoms caused by remote dissemination—bone pain, anemia, weight loss—while the prostate itself still causes no symptoms. Or the growth of the gland locally may cause the first symptoms, similar to symptoms caused by BPH; perhaps 25 percent of men who suddenly can't pee (acute retention) have prostatic cancer. Sometimes it grows rapidly. When it does appear in the young, it often seems to be more lethal, but this is uncertain.

A skilled examiner can make the diagnosis on rectal examination because the tumor feels characteristically hard, like a rock, but he confirms his diagnosis with a needle biopsy. For this, a small specimen, sucked into a needle that has been inserted into the tumor, usually by way of the rectum, is examined by a pathologist. With confirmation of the diagnosis, the examiner then takes some additional steps in order to determine the tumor's stage: special X rays such as a CAT (computer assisted tomography) scan, X rays after injections of the lymph vessels, or even an operation to find out if lymph nodes are diseased. He may not be able to make a final staging until lymph nodes removed at surgery have been examined. Because your doctor is likely to refer to the "stage," you might want to know what this means (Jewett, 1975).

Stage A: Tumor confined within the capsule (the outer covering) of the gland. A-1: Relatively benign appearing under the microscope; probably will stay where it is without spreading. A-2: On microscopic examination, appears to be a faster growing tumor. May spread. The stage A tumors cause no symptoms, and therefore will have been discovered incidentally.

Stage B: The tumor has filled and invaded the capsule of the gland, but it has extended no farther. In a survey conducted by the American College of Surgeons, 55 percent of patients with prostatic cancer had stage A or B tumors.

Stage C: The tumor has spread to adjacent tissues or organs within the pelvis.

Stage D: Distant spread, perhaps to the bones or the lungs.

INDICATIONS FOR SURGERY

Authorities who write about this disease have advised your urologist to base his recommendations for treatment on the stage of the disease. Unfortunately, however, these recommendations are on rather insecure clinical footing, because the authorities haven't yet managed to conduct adequate random, controlled clinical tests on which to base them. At any rate, it goes like this:

Stage A-1: Possibly no immediate treatment, maybe these tumors are not true cancers. You can't be sure just by looking at them under the microscope; you'd have to see what happens. They may never grow. Follow-up every three months advised. Or for young patients (anyone under sixty they call young in this league) radical prostatectomy or radiation therapy (see under "Alternatives") are considered legitimate. Even endocrine therapy is okay, particularly among the old. The problem is that no one knows who will have a very slow-growing cancer, and who will have an invasive, rapidly growing tumor. Thus, for stage A-1 your urologist can recommend just about anything that pleases him and still snuggle comfortably under the blanket of conventional dogma.

Stage A-2: Immediate definitive treatment with either radical prostatectomy or radiation. Which one? Your guess is probably about as good as your urologist's. I'll go into this later on.

Stage B: Radical prostatectomy advised for those who are acceptable surgical risks with a life expectancy of at least ten years. Or external beam radiation may be preferred. Sometimes radiation is used after the prostatectomy. Implantation of radioactive iodine or gold directly into the tumor may be an acceptable option. Thus for many patients: uncertainty as to whether surgery or radiation is best.

Stage C: Radiation therapy is probably best. Urologists have tried surgery, and it didn't work out too well. Endocrine therapy given in addition to radiation may delay the onset of distant spread, but when given early in treatment of this stage, it does not prolong overall survival.

Stage D: All types of treatment may come into play: radiation, endocrine treatment, and finally chemotherapy. Often these treatments seem to be measures of last resort, as they are for many cancers, but radiation and endocrine treatment (castration works best) have produced striking, though temporary, results.

THE OPERATION

Radical prostatectomy, first used in 1905, has become the customary operation for the cancerous prostate. The surgeon removes the entire prostate and its capsule, along with the seminal vesicles (small storage vessels for semen located where the ducts from the testicles join the urethra), through either the perineal or retropubic route (see the section on BPH surgery for description of these routes). Because removal of the seminal vesicles interrupts the flow of sperm as effectively as a vasectomy, the patient is left sterile. If, as is usually the case, the nerves that control erection are removed along with the prostate, the patient is also left impotent.

Should the operation be lifesaving, loss of sexual potency is, plainly, a secondary consideration, but the operation may not be lifesaving, its indications are unclear, and it is in competition with radiation, which doesn't cause impotency as frequently. Therefore, operating urologists have met this competitive challenge by devising a radical prostatectomy that preserves the nerves—thereby preserving sexual function, they say. In one series of sixty patients, who had been potent preoperatively and were subjected to this modification of the radical prostatectomy, from 33 percent to 84 percent (depending on the extent of tumor invasion) remained potent postoperatively (Eggleston and Walsh, 1985). Later, however, Walsh, at a consensus conference, warned that age also influences results (Barnes, 1987). Of men in their thirties all were potent after the operation, but only 14 percent of those aged seventy to seventy-nine.

RESULTS

Approximately 5 percent of patients die of radical prostatectomy surgery; from 2 percent to 57 percent suffer urinary incontinence and miscellaneous complications; after the conventional operation, about 90 percent suffer erectile impotence. Finally, tumor recurs at the operative site in from 4 percent to 22 percent.

If the disease has not spread beyond the capsule of the gland at the time of surgery (therefore a local disease—stage A-2 or B), survival statistics are excellent. In two recent series approximately 94 percent survived five years, and 86 percent of these survivors were apparently free of disease (Gibbons, 1984; Middleton, 1986). Those skeptical of surgical accomplishment have pointed out that these good results may be due to the benign natural history of local disease rather than to the effectiveness of the radical operation (Jacobi and Hohenfellner, 1982). Local disease, easy to cure or permanently local in any case, favorably biases the results of its treatment. In England most patients with small, local tumors have limited surgery merely to relieve the obstruction rather than radical prostatectomy; after which they are left alone (Barnes, 1987).

We once more face a profound lack of good data. No one has carried out controlled clinical tests comparing radical prostatectomy for local disease with lesser treatments or with no treatment. A hope for the future, some urologists say, but such tests are expensive and slow; fulfillment of that hope seems unlikely.

When the surgeon intends to relieve obstruction and not attempt cure (in stage C or D), TURP, the operation employed for BPH, may be used, often along with hormones. Because any one of them will suppress the production of male hormone—known to promote growth of the cancer—castration (the most effective), adrenalectomy (removal of one or both adrenal glands), or hypophysectomy (removal of the pituitary) have been used.

ALTERNATIVES

After a Veterans Administration study (1967) showed that hormone treatment didn't cure the disease, radiotherapists went to work. As a result radiation has become the best alternative to radical prostatectomy. Although the cancer is only moderately radiosensitive, the radiotherapists hit it hard with carefully focused, high-voltage machines or with direct implantations to obtain good results with minimal postoperative sexual impotence, at least in local disease. Survival at ten years is similar to that of radical prostatectomy; unclear still, however, is the relative success of surgery and radiation in producing lifelong freedom from recurrence (Resnick, 1989). Therapy lasts for seven to eight weeks, five days a week.

A random, controlled clinical test comparing surgery and radiation would help everybody concerned—you in particular if you're going to have to decide what treatment you want. But, as I said, no such test is in the works. In any case, I don't think such a test would reveal much difference between surgery and radiation. It's probably a toss-up.

In the 1940s Charles Huggins (1941) demonstrated convincingly that hormone treatment could shrink the cancer. I still remember our original incredulity when this rather nervous man (he kept plucking at his wristwatch band) displayed before-and-after X rays on the viewbox. Could we believe the almost complete disappearance of bony spread shown in the after films? We scrutinized the dates on the films to make sure their order was correct—can't fudge film dates. It turned out that Charles Huggins was right; his work confirmed, he was awarded the Nobel Prize for medicine in 1966.

Unfortunately, hormonal treatment failed to cure the disease. The Veterans Administration study (1967) compared radical prostatectomy and estrogen therapy and concluded that estrogen therapy increases the risk of death from heart disease or stroke. They found little clinical benefit from either castration (orchiectomy) or a daily dose of female hormones unless the cancer had spread distantly and was causing serious problems. Today hormone therapy is reserved for patients with advanced disease (stage C or D) and severe symptoms. Either estrogen alone or orchiectomy alone provides all of the benefits of both combined, but with estrogen 20 percent of patients have died of cardiovascular complications (Lytton 1988); castration doesn't include this risk. If afflicted with severe pain from spread to bones, patients with advanced disease are usually willing to give up their testicles for relief, but a gonadotropin-releasing hormone may prove to be as effective in hormone-sensitive disease.

As with many advanced cancers, chemotherapy may come into use for cancer of the prostate, but it doesn't help much, and it brings with it many side effects.

7

Cesarean Section

Kate T., a thirty-six-year-old mother of a five-year-old boy and three-year-old girl, now in the ninth month of her third pregnancy, felt a sharp pain in her lower abdomen at noon Thursday. When this recurred about thirty minutes later, she went to the hospital, where they observed her for a couple of hours and then sent her home. "Sorry, dear, false labor."

After a restless night, she awoke at 6 A.M. Now she knew she was in labor; it felt just like it had with Bonnie, her second child. The nurses in the obstetrical unit were still doubtful at first, but they kept her there. Soon the pains became more regular, and at about 11 A.M. her waters broke.

"How is . . . it?" asked Kate.

"Fine," said the nurse as she changed Kate's sheet.

"What's that green stuff?"

"That's a little meconium, but don't worry. The doctor's coming." The nurse fastened electrodes to Kate's abdomen to monitor the baby's heart rate. Kate remembered that meconium is the fetal stool, and when it came out early, it may be a sign of fetal distress.

During her examination the doctor applied an electrode to the infant's scalp, which was accessible through the mouth of the womb. The doctor and the nurses—and Kate too—could now count the baby's heart rate. As the labor wore on, they gave her epidural anesthesia (nerve injection at the tailbone) to reduce the pain and pitocin to increase the strength of her contractions, but she made little progress.

The baby's heart rate slowed, whereupon the nurses gave Kate oxygen and turned her on her left side. The heart rate increased. An hour later it slowed again.

"If you want to operate, that's all right with me," said Kate. "I don't want to hurt her . . . I mean the baby."

The doctor, who had returned to the labor room and examined her, said, "Don't worry, Kate. There's no reason to do a cesarean section now. Everything is all right. You're dilating nicely." She held Kate's hand for a few moments. Kate wondered how the doctor, mother of an eight-year-old boy, had had it with her own labor. Not as bad as this labor, she bet.

Every time she had a contraction, the baby's heart rate slowed. An hour after the doctor's last visit when Kate was convinced that she was getting nowhere, she spoke to the nurse again: "How long are you going to wait? I'm not getting anywhere, am I? And the kid is probably suffocating. You ought to operate and take it out, shouldn't you?"

"It's up to Dr. Worth, you know. She knows what's going on."

Finally, Kate felt the kind of strong contractions she remembered from her last labor. She was at last fully dilated. At 7:30 P.M. the doctor arrived and delivered a healthy boy.

Cesarean section had not been necessary, might not even have been considered except for the monitoring. The doctor showed Kate how the umbilical cord had passed around the baby's neck; perhaps during labor traction on the cord had reduced the circulation and caused the heart rate to drop. They gave Kate some more epidural anesthesia, and, by prior agreement, the doctor ligated Kate's tubes. Kate would have no more of this.

She had avoided what, it turns out, would have been an unnecessary cesarean section, but many young mothers don't avoid it. At 911,000 a year, cesarean section has become the most frequent hospital-based operation in the United States (U.S. Department of Health and Human Services, 1986). Medical and lay authorities agree: Safe cesarean section, a great achievement of twentieth-century medicine, is now used far too often. Currently the most shocking surgical excess, half the cesarean sections done may be unnecessary. The profession has failed in self-control. You'll have to take responsibility.

If you are in the hands of an obstetrician whom you respect with the tense situation of a labor already begun, you may find it difficult to challenge the recommendation of a cesarean section. Maybe, like Kate, you'll even ask to have one. But you might want to know how critical the indications are, and if you are not convinced, then ask for a delay. Of course you'll feel more comfortable with the issue if you have discussed it with your doctor beforehand—something this chapter hopes to prepare you for.

The principal objections to its excessive use are greater injury to the mother when compared to vaginal delivery and cost. Are infants better off with cesarean section? In some cases, yes, but obstetricians don't know with sufficient precision in just which cases.

Faced with this lack of adequate medical certainty and the threat of malpractice suits unless they do "everything" to avoid fetal risk, obstetricians will doubtless continue to overuse cesarean section. If you want to avoid having this operation unnecessarily, you'll have to criticize, and possibly oppose, your doctor's recommendation, and maybe your own inclinations, intelligently.

HISTORY

The name "cesarean" has been credited to the belief that Julius Caesar entered the world this way. Not likely, however, because Julius Caesar's mother survived his entry into middle age, and in the time of Caesar the operation was done only on dead mothers—live babies from dead mothers—if it were done at all (Wangensteen, 1978). Possibly the word is derived from the Latin verb *caedere*, "to cut" (Prichard et al., 1985).

The first authentic case of a live baby extracted surgically from a live mother occurred in 1610 in Wittenberg, Germany. In the following two and a half centuries doctors performed the operation rarely—for good reason: They had catastrophic results. In the middle of the last century, major hospitals had to admit to appalling maternal mortality rates for cesarean section—85 to 100 percent.

Asepsis, anesthesia, better techniques, intravenous fluids, blood transfusions, antibiotics, and other refinements of modern medicine dramatically changed this outcome during the twentieth century. Maternal mortality fell to below 1 per 1,000. Obstetricians finally began to use the operation with confidence. In 1963 a hospital reported that cesarean section had been used in 3.3 percent of its deliveries—thought to be a reasonable incidence at the time (Wangensteen, 1978).

FREQUENCY

But during the 1970s the cesarean birth rate shot up to reach 15.2 percent of deliveries nationwide. By 1984 the rate had increased to 21.1 percent for a yearly total of 814,000, and by 1986 to 24.1 percent and 911,000 (U.S. Department of Health and Human Services 1986). Cesarean section had suddenly become the most frequent operation in this country.

The rate is increasing in every country, but with sharp national differences (Notzon et al., 1987). In Czechoslovakia, for instance, the rate is only 5 percent. We have the highest rate, with Canada second. Some analysts have defended these high rates by pointing out that the rate of infant deaths at the time of delivery (perinatal mortality) has fallen as the rate for C-section has risen; thus liberal use of C-section may have saved infant lives. But countries with lower perinatal mortality rates than the United States also have lower C-section rates, and many innovations in prenatal and newborn care, independent of cesarean section, have worked to reduce perinatal mortality.

Professional and public concern with the astonishing increase in cesarean-section frequency led to a NIH consensus development task force (1980), which formulated recommendations that were expected to lead to a decrease in the national rates. Didn't work; rates continued to rise. The most recent data on rate show no evidence of even a leveling. As has often been the case, the advice of experts, academicians, and consensus conferences has not affected the behavior of practitioners.

MEDICAL EXPLANATIONS

What has happened? Why so many C-sections? The NIH consensus conference (1980) identified liberalization of surgical indications as the principal medical reason. Most of the cesarean sections are done for one of these indications: dystocia, previous cesarean birth, breech presentation, or fetal distress.

Dystocia: Dystocia means abnormal labor or abnormal childbirth. It is a grab bag of sometimes precise, sometimes vague indications: cephalopelvic disproportion (head too big for the opening), failure to progress in labor, or uterine inertia (tired womb?) are examples. We may describe the obstetrician's frequent use of this indication to justify the operation by saying that his goals are undamaged infants and a reasonable duration of labor in contrast to the older goal of eventual vaginal delivery. But it may also mean that if the obstetrician feels things have just gone on too long, if it's getting too late in the day or too near the weekend, he can, without criticism, declare dystocia and extract the infant quickly with his knife.

Previous cesarean birth: Three years ago, at the age of thirty, Sally A. delivered her first child, a nine-pound boy, by cesarean section under the care of her brother-in-law, an obstetrician. The labor had simply gone on too long, and the baby was thought to be perhaps a little too large for Sally's pelvis. After twenty hours of labor with inadequate progress, Sally readily agreed to a C-section.

Now she was pregnant again, and she and her husband, a respiratory therapist, had talked it over. They had heard about the advantage of natural childbirth. Her best friend had recently had a baby and spoke of the marvelous experience and how it had "bonded" her to her baby. Sally wanted to try. They had moved away from Portland where her first baby had been born and now lived in Palo Alto where they had a different obstetrician. After this obstetrician obtained her former medical record from Sally's brother-in-law, he agreed to try natural labor. Following an intense nine-hour labor Sally delivered a ten-pound girl vaginally. Mother and daughter both in excellent condition.

Cases such as Sally's are the exception in the United States, and previous cesarean birth has become the indication for about one third of C-sections. According to best estimates, between 30 percent and 60 percent of women with previous cesarean births could deliver vaginally, as Sally did, but in this country only 5 percent actually do. Obstetricians have followed the dictum: "Once a section always a section," but the dictum is not universally applied. In Norway, for example, 43 percent of women with previous cesarean births deliver vaginally, and their C-section rate is half that of ours.

Breech presentation: When the baby is located in the womb so that his rear end, rather than his head (the usual leading part), will come out first, obstetricians now usually recommend a cesarean section. Inasmuch as vaginal breech delivery has been accompanied by significant infant and maternal morbidity, this indication seems reasonable. Some say that vaginal breech delivery may disappear. But older obstetricians deplore the possibility that obstetricians now in training will never learn its techniques, and others call cesarean section for breech presentation a "holy cow" of obstetrical practice.

Fetal distress: This is a judgment call. If the baby seems to be getting in trouble, best not to wait. Take it out through the abdomen. But how does the obstetrician tell when the baby is in trouble? The problem has been overdiagnosis, attributable largely to electronic monitoring, a diagnostic technique with a high false-positive rate. That is to say, when the electronic monitoring suggests trouble, there may really be no trouble. Birth could proceed normally. In one controlled study, universal electronic monitoring, compared to selective monitoring of just high-risk cases, led to more C-sections, but with no improvement in results. Use it only in high-risk cases (patients with high blood pressure, breech presentation, twins, low weight fetuses, diabetes, heart trouble, infection, etc.) they concluded. Monitoring when not needed, some have pointed out, may cause such distress to the mother, that it *creates* dystocia—the most frequent indication for a C-section.

Other traditional, and acceptable, medical indications for C-section, such as a placenta blocking the way out (placenta previa), herpes, diabetes, and preeclampsia (a disease of pregnancy characterized by high blood pressure and kidney trouble) have not been responsible for the recent increased use of the operation (Bottoms et al., 1980).

NONMEDICAL EXPLANATIONS

Dr. S. F. Bottoms (1980) and other writers looking into the matter have identified several nonmedical causes for the exploitation of cesarean section. One is a changed obstetrical population that needs more C-sections: More women are having a first child, and more older women are having babies.

Another is a changed economic status that promotes more surgery. Today most patients are treated as private patients, and private patients have always had more cesarean sections. One study, for instance, found that private patients had 2.48 times as many cesarean sections as clinic patients in the same hospital, with no improvement in outcome provided by the surgery (Haynes de Regt et al., 1986). If their fees are paid for by third-party payers (medical insurance), insured patients can ignore the increased expense of a surgical delivery.

That most deliveries take place in large hospitals favors C-sections. Surgery happens readily and frequently there—usually at lower risk than in small hospitals. As the operation has become relatively safe for the mother and infant, that fact alone encourages its use.

With his patient in a large hospital where a trained crew of helpers and much shiny equipment are waiting, the obstetrician will find the convenience of a C-section alluring. Maybe he can reach home in time for dinner after all, rather than hang around after dark or get up in the middle of the night to drive back. A hard life. Specialists in obstetrics and gynecology often give up obstetrics when they get older.

While they are still in practice, obstetricians don't all practice in the same way. Style of practice is an important determinant. A study from Detroit showed that whether or not a woman has a C-section depends more on who her doctor is than on other criteria (Goyert et al., 1989). Among eleven doctors in a community hospital, the C-section rate varied from 1 in 10 to 1 in 3. Babies delivered surgically didn't do any better than the others.

Money counts too, though no one can accurately reckon its impact. Both the hospital and the doctor make more money from a cesarean section than from a normal delivery, and they both think they need more money. If he hopes to pay his burgeoning malpractice premiums, the obstetrician surely needs money. Said one discouraged obstetrician, "It's like paying the salary of a third person. There's me, my partner, and the malpractice premium."

LEGAL ISSUES

Only neurosurgeons are sued more often than obstetricians. Three quarters of the members of the American College of Obstetrics and Gynecology have been sued for malpractice at least once. They hate it. It raises their premiums, damages their reputation, injures their pride, and destroys their practice. So they fight back, try to protect themselves. In Brunswick, Georgia, obstetricians have counterattacked by refusing to care for women malpractice lawyers or the wives or associates of such lawyers (Cooke, 1987). This warfare may spread.

They also defend themselves with cesarean sections. If the baby doesn't turn out to be perfect, and some don't, no matter what is done (the defect may be congenital or in other ways beyond a physician's control), the obstetrician fears that he may be sued, especially if he hasn't done "everything"—including a C-section. He feels safer by using surgery on slight pretext. The obstetrician's need to protect himself against malpractice may be the chief nonmedical cause for the overuse of cesarean section.

THE OPERATION

Under general, spinal, or regional anesthesia, through an up-and-down or crosswise incision in the lower abdomen, the surgeon enters the abdominal cavity (Prichard et al., 1985). The uterus, by now very prominent, is separated from the bladder and opened, usually with a transverse incision because it provides a stronger scar than a vertical incision, just enough to allow delivery of the fetal head—the largest diameter of a newborn baby. As the shoulder appears, the mother is given oxytocin, a drug which causes the uterus to contract, thereby simplifying delivery of the rest of the baby and the placenta (the afterbirth). Because the baby's exit provides so much extra space, the incisions in the uterus and abdominal wall are easily closed. The mother is allowed to get up and around soon after surgery.

RESULTS, RISKS, AND COMPLICATIONS

The risks of C-section are mostly to the mother. Maternal mortality is 10.8 per 10,000 as compared with only 1.7 per 10,000 for vaginal delivery (Minkoff and Schwarz, 1980). Postoperative morbidity is about ten times more frequent for C-section; it comprises the usual complications of abdominal surgery: wound infection, hemorrhage, thrombophlebitis (inflamed veins), pneumonia, emboli (circulating blood clots), wound hernia, bladder infection, etc.

Most fetal death and damage at the time of delivery is unpreventable, whether or not C-section is used, because it results from earlier events uncontrollable by the physician. But some fetal death and damage at the time of delivery is preventable by the reasonable use of cesarean section for the medical indications I have mentioned above. The operation doesn't always succeed, of course. As might be expected, the infant mortality rate (perinatal mortality rate) associated with C-section is higher than that associated with vaginal delivery.

Overall, the perinatal mortality rate has dropped as the cesarean section rate has increased, and this has been taken as justification for liberal use of the operation. As I pointed out earlier, however, perinatal mortality rates are less in several European countries where the C-section rate remains lower than it does here, and many beneficial changes in obstetrical and pediatric practice have come into play simultaneously with increased use of C-section. Freer C-section application may have played little or no role in reducing perinatal mortality. Speculation defines the debate, not sound data.

The question might be resolved, I suppose, by setting up a random, controlled clinical test in which cesarean section was compared with vaginal delivery for the borderline indications that are presently the cause of so many operations. You would think, moreover, that responsibility for proof would be with those who are doing a great volume of surgical deliveries, but its patrons are neither now undertaking nor soon apt to undertake a controlled clinical test of C-section.

A SENSIBLE PROGRAM

Obstetricians are much aware of their critics both within and without the specialty. Many are trying to spread the word and slow the carnage, but professional education hasn't done the job. Maybe tough hospital controls of physician behavior will help. Stephen A. Myers and Norbert Gleicher (1988) report success with such a program at Mount Sinai Hospital in Chicago. With voluntary physician participation in their program, the cesarean section rate fell from 17.5 percent in 1985 to 11.5 percent in 1987.

The program included a stringent requirement for a second opinion, use of objective criteria for the four most common indications for cesarean section, a detailed review of all cesarean sections, and a review of individual physicians' rates of performing them. Women who had previously undergone cesarean section must be allowed to try a vaginal delivery; fetuses in breech presentation should in most cases undergo vaginal delivery (this is rarely done in most hospitals); a diagnosis of failure to progress in labor could be made only after a woman had made no progress for at least two hours of regular contractions; and fetal distress could be diagnosed only if the child's heart rate and blood chemistries confirmed the diagnosis. Does your hospital practice similar controls? Perhaps it should.

ALTERNATIVES

You might avoid an unnecessary operation by talking the problem over with your obstetrician before labor. Speak your mind. Normal vaginal delivery is the obvious alternative, and your obstetrician, who is no doubt sensitive to the criticism, may quite easily be persuaded toward vaginal delivery if you yourself favor it.

Maybe it's a matter of trying for a vaginal delivery after a previous C-section. About 50 percent can make it with a "trial of labor" (Shiono et al., 1987). If you let your obstetrician know you are aware of that, he might reign in his surgical impulsiveness a bit. Here's another example: You may not need electronic monitoring (Leveno et al., 1986). It overdiagnoses trouble and results in unnecessary surgery. Think about what's going on. Take responsibility. Complete trust in your physician may seem ideal, but the present medical climate doesn't justify it.

HOME DELIVERY—MIDWIVES

By the time you have had a recommendation for a cesarean section, it's too late for you to think about having a home delivery. Because your medical insurance covers hospital costs, you might never have thought about it. Why bother? Still . . . those who have experienced it say that home delivery, aided by a nurse-midwife, will bring you, your mate, and your family far closer to the marvelous process of birth than a hospital delivery. Further, it is an alternative that will probably raise your chances of evading unnecessary surgery. Trained midwives are quick to refer complicated cases to an obstetrician, but equivocal cases are less likely to be rushed to surgery. If there is time, or perhaps for a later pregnancy, or for advice to a friend, you might want to consider home delivery—provided that you can find someone to help you carry it out. It's neither common in most parts of this country nor popular with the medical profession.

Because it takes a lot of professional time, doctors have found home delivery inefficient and no safer for the mother and child than hospital delivery. In the middle of the nineteenth century it *was* safer, then in the earlier part of this century less safe than hospital care, now probably about as safe. Doctors are no longer trained to carry it out, however. Northwestern Medical School, where I worked, closed its once-thriving Chicago Maternity Center Home Delivery Service (created to teach general practitioners the art) years ago; the story has been the same for other medical schools.

In most developed countries, home deliveries now make up less than 2 percent of births. As an exception, the Netherlands has one third of its deliveries at home. For them it works. They report a total cesarean section rate, including both hospital and home deliveries, of only 5 percent and a low perinatal mortality rate.

While modern doctors have abandoned home delivery, trained nurse-midwives, in the revival of an ancient craft, have taken it up. Although experienced women have always helped the novice with her birthing, formal training for midwives was started by Hippocrates in the fifth century B.C. (Speert, 1986). Mostly, throughout history however, it has been a self-taught skill, or one passed on by older midwives who were in control. It took male physicians a long time to move in on the midwives. In 1552 Wertt, a physician in Hamburg, was burned at the stake for having posed as a woman in order to attend a delivery. As late as the eighteenth century physicians were rarely summoned for childbirth, and at the beginning of this century, in 1909, 3,000 New York City midwives still handled 40 percent of the deliveries. But by 1956 the turnover was complete, fourteen midwives performed only 142 deliveries in New York. Man—for doctors were almost all men—had, in an odd, indirect way, finally extricated the process of birth from woman and called it his own.

Man hasn't given it up, of course, but women are now on the way back. In what has been called a "feminization of the specialty" OB/GYN residencies currently attract a larger proportion of women than before (Jonas, 1987), and a lively and competent group of well-trained nurse-midwives have almost replaced the "granny" midwives of old. These nurse-midwives now number about 2,000 in the United States. Some practice as private nurse-midwives with hospital deliveries or as obstetrician-nurses; or they may practice in hospitals for the indigent, in freestanding birth centers, or in health maintenance organizations; finally, they may carry out home births. Home births, however, account for no more than about 1 percent of the national birth total (Rooks and Haas, 1986). It's something you may want, but you'll have to search for it. Your OB specialist is not apt to recommend it.

8

Hysterectomy

Hysterectomy, at 636,000 a year the second most frequent hospital-based operation in the United States, ranks just behind cesarean section. When it peaked in 1975, before cesarean section had accelerated to pass it, it ranked first. If surgeons had continued operating at their 1975 rate, 62 percent of all American women would have lost their wombs by age seventy (Sandberg et al., 1985)—to a usually fruitless surgical assault. But now, perhaps because of citizen's complaints and the profession's embarrassed response, surgeons have slowed down a bit. Many physicians, third-party payers, feminists, consumer groups, and government agencies have complained about its overuse. The pace has eased off but it's still a vastly overused operation.

One evening in late November Maria K., a sixty-five-year-old widow, arrived at the emergency room, vomiting. She said it had started early in the morning, cramps first and then the vomiting, and now she couldn't keep anything down. She had passed nothing through her rectum for twenty-four hours. Her abdomen, scarred from several previous operations, was distended; her urine was concentrated, and her red blood cell count high, indicating severe dehydration. X rays showed a small bowel filled with gas but no gas in the large bowel. The diagnosis was intestinal obstruction, probably due to old postoperative adhesions.

After inserting tubes into her stomach and bladder and hydrating her with intravenous fluids, Dr. C., the general surgeon on call, opened her abdomen at 1 A.M., and in a difficult and hazardous procedure (spillage of fluid from an obstructed bowel caused by a nick in the bowel can be fatal) divided the adhesions that produced the obstruction.

On Friday, two days later, the case was discussed at grand rounds. "Most of the adhesions were deep in the pelvis," said Dr. C., "at the site of her hysterectomy. Of course, she had some adhesions in her upper abdomen too, the site of her cholecystectomy, and then before that she'd had a partial gastrectomy, but those adhesions weren't causing the obstruction."

"How many belly operations has she had?" asked a staff surgeon.

Dr. C. gestured to Dr. T., the surgical resident on the case. "It's hard to be sure," the resident said. "She's a little vague herself. But the gallbladder, the gastric resection—for ulcer it seems—the hysterectomy, for I don't know what, at least two previous operations for adhesions—all of these at other hospitals—and something about an exploratory laparotomy for a displaced kidney. We don't know much about that. Oh, yes, there was a wound hernia too, about five years ago. And a face lift, I forgot that, but I don't know about anything else."

"She sounds like one of those people who shop around from one hospital to another, collecting operations," said the staff surgeon. "She'll go some place else next time. What is it? . . . Munchhausen syndrome? No? Or polysurgery . . . I think. Menninger, the psychiatrist, called it that—addicted to surgery. Like any other addiction, I guess, but probably more dangerous. I read someplace that polysurgery seems to be getting more common."

Dr. C. grunted, signaling impatience, but the staff surgeon continued: "They seem to be willing anyway. Trouble is that they can afford it now that their insurance covers any damn thing they want." This staff surgeon, older than the others, was considered a skeptic, even a cynic at times.

"But *this* operation couldn't be avoided," claimed Dr. C. "She really was obstructed."

"Sure, I know, but did she need the hysterectomy that caused the trouble?" asked the staff surgeon. Dr. C. shrugged, unknowing.

It was touch and go with Maria for five days, until she started passing gas through her rectum, but she recovered. Before she left the hospital, she asked the resident to look and see if her tonsils had grown back. Her throat had been sore, she said. She wondered if she needed to have them taken out again.

Hysterectomy is done too frequently and for indications too vague and controversial. If your doctor has recommended it for you, think about it. Make sure you need it, and consider the information in this chapter. Most hysterectomies are done on women in their reproductive years when, you would think, they might still have use for a womb.

Doctors fail to agree on hysterectomy's indications. Whether they recommend it or not depends, among other odd things, upon where you live. If, for example, you live in the South or the West, you are more apt to have the operation recommended to you than if you live in the Northeast, although the gynecological character of the population seems to be about the same in those locations (Dicker et al., 1982). Such variations in incidence depend more on the supply of surgeons and their style of surgical practice than on the real need of their patients.

INDICATIONS

The needs of their patients are variously understood by surgeons. Stated opinions range from those requiring, sensibly it seems to me, that hysterectomy shouldn't be undertaken unless there is something definitely wrong with the organ, "hysterectomy," they say "in the absence of pelvic disease cannot be justified any more than can removal of the normal breast or gallbladder," to opinion that may advocate removal whether it's abnormal or not. "Pathologic alteration (disease) in the uterus is frequently irrelevant to the indication for hysterectomy today," say these aggressive surgeons (Esterday, et al., 1983). For them almost anything goes.

For a few major problems, however, gynecologists do agree. For cancer, for life-threatening infection, or for some of the immediate complications of pregnancy, such as a ruptured uterus, the indications for hysterectomy are compelling. Cancer of the body of the uterus (endometrial cancer) is an absolute indication for the operation; cancer of the mouth of the uterus (the cervix) is a relative indication. If detected early by the well-known Pap smear, cancer of the cervix can be treated by local excision; more advanced stages require hysterectomy or radiotherapy.

At one end of the spectrum of medical indications—where there are the indications I have just listed—we find agreement. At the other end—hysterectomy in order to prevent conditions that may never occur—we find intense disagreement. In between, either hysterectomy or its alternatives may reasonably be advocated.

A study reported from the Harvard School of Public Health found 92 percent of hysterectomies performed for reasons other than those upon which there is medical agreement (Sandberg et al., 1985). They are performed for benign tumors (myomas), dysfunctional uterine bleeding (abnormal menstruation), or pelvic relaxation (dropping down of the uterus and other late, weak-muscle complications of childbirth). Sometimes the uterus is removed incidentally when the ovaries and tubes are being removed for infection, or it is removed for endometriosis (see below), or merely for sterilization—rarely justified. At cesarean section, for example, hysterectomy is not justified for other than conditions such as cancer or hemorrhage from an unextractable placenta (placenta accreta), that would justify hysterectomy independently of the desire for sterilization.

MYOMA

Twenty percent (higher in blacks) of women over thirty-five harbor uterine myomas (Entman, 1988). Most of these benign tumors (also called leiomyomas or fibroids), which are made of the same smooth muscle as the uterus itself with some added fibrous tissue, need never be removed. They grow slowly; if multiple they produce a lumpy uterus. Rarely, they reach the size of a full-term fetus. Their cause is unknown, but in order to grow they do require female hormones. As a consequence, they shrink after menopause and are less frequent in older women.

The diagnosis is made by pelvic examination, by D and C (scraping out of the uterus), by laparoscopy (a look through a tube inserted inside the abdomen through the abdominal wall), by ultrasonography (diagnostic technique using high frequency sound waves), by CAT scan (computer assisted tomography), or at surgery. If they cause you no symptoms, don't worry about them. The risk-benefit ratio of hysterectomy for asymptomatic myomas of different estimated sizes and weights is unknown. Hence rigid size criteria (for example: if big as a twelve-week fetus, take it out) are not sound indications. The usual indications for surgery are pain or excessive menstrual bleeding due to the myomas, but a causal relationship between the myomas and the symptoms supposedly attributed to them may be uncertain. Pain and bleeding have many causes, and in any case, the indications, even with related symptoms, are not compelling. Myomas are not life-threatening; occasionally hysterectomy does threaten life.

Alternatives to hysterectomy for myoma are excision of the individual tumors (occasionally done if there are only one or two), or simply neglect. After menopause myomas stop appearing, and the old ones shrink.

DYSFUNCTIONAL UTERINE BLEEDING

Abnormal bleeding usually has a cause. Myomas are one cause, incomplete abortion another; endometriosis (see below), polyps, vaginitis, ovarian disease, blood diseases, etc., may cause bleeding. The gynecologist may encounter someone with excessive or long-lasting menstrual bleeding who has none of these clear organic causes; this he may then designate as "dysfunctional bleeding." It's a loose term and refers to bleeding caused by a failure in the way that the ovaries and the uterine lining are coordinated functionally. Normal menstrual bleeding is hormonally controlled, but sometimes menstruation doesn't stop as quickly as it should. Near the menarche (beginning of menstruation) or the menopause (its end) a failure of the ovary to produce an ovum (the egg) regularly may upset the hormonal control.

No matter what the cause, the experience of heavy menstrual bleeding time after time can be nerve-racking, and a victim can lose enough blood to cause anemia. Dysfunctional uterine bleeding has become an important indication for hysterectomy.

However, most gynecologists would agree that hysterectomy should be considered only after curettage (D and C—scraping out the womb) plus hormonal treatment have failed to control the bleeding. How many times should curettage be tried? Matter of judgment, of course, but don't be in a hurry to try something more radical. Menopause will naturally bring the bleeding to an end, and so will pregnancy.

PELVIC RELAXATION

Vaginal relaxation and uterine prolapse (the uterus falling down from its normal position, possibly as far as the vaginal opening) account for 30 percent to 40 percent of vaginal hysterectomies (Burnett, L.S., 1988).

Normally the uterus is located above the vagina, between the bladder and the rectum, with its opening, the cervix, protruding about an inch into the vagina. Following childbirth when it shrinks, the uterus may fail to move back up to its normal position, particularly if there is a genetic predisposition to pelvic relaxation. Muscles of the pelvic floor no longer hold the organs in their best locations: The uterus slips down into the vagina (prolapse), sometimes bringing the back wall of the bladder or the front wall of the rectum down with it (cystocele or rectocele). A dragging discomfort, backache, and urinary incontinence (stress incontinence) may follow.

In order to help make a technically strong repair (a colporrhaphy) of the relaxed pelvis, gynecologists will remove the uterus. Whether or not you decide to accept the operation will depend upon how severely the symptoms of prolapse trouble you. Obviously you don't want it if you intend to have more children. A minimum age limit for colporrhaphy of thirty to forty-five years has been proposed—but generally ignored.

If your symptoms are mild, exercises may strengthen the pelvic floor so that you can avoid surgery, and as another alternative, a pessary will hold up almost any dropped womb. It's a doughnut-shaped, and almost doughnut-sized, device that the gynecologist places in the vagina, where it remains until the next time you go in for cleansing and replacement. You might not want to deal with this kind of thing permanently, but it could be a good alternative to surgery until you have completed your family.

Women have accepted hysterectomy for the benign condition called endometriosis, in which fragments of the uterine lining, the endometrium, are spilled out into the pelvic cavity—probably by passing out through the fallopian tubes. The fragments irritate surrounding tissue to produce adhesions and scars, which cause pain and infertility. In extreme cases this disease may require hysterectomy and removal of the tubes and ovaries. Relatively mild cases are treated with hormones or with local surgery to remove the displaced endometrial fragments.

QUALITY OF LIFE

Many women have had hysterectomy to prevent something unwanted—pregnancy, say—or to avoid something feared—cancer, say—and thereby achieve what is now popularly called an improved "quality of life." Depends upon what you need for the quality of your life, I guess. As many as one out of five hysterectomies have been done principally to prevent pregnancy. The technique is at least unquestionably effective. To reasonable minds, however, this is "like cracking a nut with a sledgehammer." Hysterectomy is not indicated for sterilization unless uterine pathology—an incipient cancer (cancer in situ), for example—would justify the operation. Don't submit to hysterectomy, a major operation, when a tubal ligation through a laparoscope (the instrument, mentioned earlier, that is inserted into the abdomen through a small incision) will effectively attain sterilization.

With your uterus removed, you will, clearly, never acquire a cancer of the uterus, but does major surgery to prevent a relatively uncommon cancer make sense? Hysterectomy as prophylaxis? If the tubes and ovaries are removed at the same time, you will avoid ovarian cancer. (The breasts then to evade breast cancer?) With your ovaries gone, you will need ovarian-hormone pills—a lifetime on pills—or without pills you will risk early cardiovascular disease. Unpleasant prospects. If however, a uterine-cancer family history puts you in a high risk group, you might consider it nonetheless, particularly if you want no more children and have other possible indications for hysterectomy, such as myomas or pelvic relaxation. But if a fear of cancer is your only reason for wanting the surgery, perhaps you should seek psychological help rather than a surgeon.

THE OPERATION

Surgeons reach the uterus by way of the abdomen or the vagina (Burnett, 1988). An incision in the lower abdomen, similar to that used for a cesarean section, allows removal of big myomas and an easier removal of the tubes and ovaries, should this be necessary, than does a vaginal hysterectomy. It turns out, incidentally, that the ovaries are removed in about a quarter of hysterectomies. At one time, the cervix might have been left behind and only the body of the uterus removed, but now the cervix is removed too—as cancer prophylaxis, they say.

About one fourth of hysterectomies are done vaginally, that is, from below through the vaginal orifice. The cervix of the uterus is separated from the vaginal wall and the uterus is pulled down into the vagina and detached. Though an individual surgeon may prefer one route or the other (doctors deliver the kinds of services they are trained to deliver), for routine cases of uterine prolapse or pelvic relaxation the vaginal route is generally favored. A repair of the pelvic floor, at the same operation, may follow the hysterectomy.

When cancer is the indication, the approach is abdominal, to allow what is called a "radical" hysterectomy—radical because more is taken out. In addition to taking out the uterus, the tubes, and the ovaries, the surgeon resects (removes part of) the lymph nodes, other tissues adjacent to the uterus, and the upper part of the vagina—all this in order to get beyond the margins of the cancer.

BENEFITS, COSTS, AND RISKS

The benefits of a hysterectomy for the benign conditions I have discussed are effective sterilization (remember, however, that tubal ligation is safer and easier), elimination of a cancer risk, and possibly an improved "quality of life."

The immediate risks are operative mortality—about 1 in a 1,000—and postoperative complications, about 1 in 4. Fever and hemorrhage are the most common complications. Late costs are inability to bear children, increased risk of coronary heart disease, early menopause, psychological depression, loss of the perception of femininity for some, and the late complications of any abdominal operation (adhesions as in the case of Maria K., for example). If the ovaries and fallopian tubes have been left behind, you may incur the "residual ovary syndrome" (abdominal pain, painful coitus, and a pelvic mass). If, on the other hand, your ovaries are removed, you'll have to take hormones. Financial costs are noteworthy: In this country we spend over $1.7 billion a year on hysterectomies (Esterday et al., 1983).

Cost–benefit scholars, to whom elimination of a cancer risk counts as an important benefit and operative mortality as an important cost, try to determine the possible usefulness of hysterectomy. In an example of such studies, Sonja Sandberg and her associates (1985), using a complex analysis, concluded that a hysterectomy in a forty-year-old woman would, because of its cancer-sparing, add 0.01 years of life on the average and 0.07 years if the ovaries were removed as well. When you consider that it takes longer than 0.07 years to recover from an uncomplicated operation, this doesn't add up to much benefit on the average. These studies don't, by the way, put a value on the psychological effects of the loss of a uterus.

"Neither prevention of cancer nor contraceptive sterilization appears to justify elective hysterectomy in healthy women," was the conclusion of a special committee of the American College of Obstetricians and Gyne-cologists (Esterday et al., 1983). Further, they argued against the use of elective hysterectomy for asymptomatic women. As is usually the case with an overused operation, the opinion proclaimed by traditional authorities comes out on the side of caution and common sense. Organized, academic medicine usually tries to support your best interests. The breakdown of good intentions occurs in the medical marketplace.

STRATEGIES TO ELIMINATE UNNECESSARY HYSTERECTOMIES

Peer review and second opinions are two strategies recommended to eliminate unnecessary hysterectomies. Unless your insurance company forces you to obtain a second opinion and pays for it, you will bear the responsibility for procuring it—more about this in Chapter 19. Your doctors and the medical establishment bear the responsibility for peer review. Here the idea is for the doctors in a hospital to check up on one another and punish, or slap wrists, or at least point out deviations from good practice. In the better hospitals, regular clinical conferences, during which cases with complications are reviewed in open discussion and doctors have to defend and explain what they have done or intend to do, are the major peer-review effort.

Tissue committees that examine surgical specimens and thereby judge whether or not operations were suitable form another arm of the peer-review effort. No doubt, as surgeon Mark Ravitch has said, "The lowest mortality and fewest complications result from the removal of normal organs." But tissue committees oppose that scandal. Their ideal: Surgeons should take out only diseased organs. This ideal breaks down, unfortunately, in the case of hysterectomy—as it does for many types of surgery—because the uterus in cases of dysfunctional bleeding or prolapse, for which the surgery may truly be justified, usually shows no discernible pathology. Thus, any normal uterus may slip through their critical net. They can't tell if the operation was justified or not. Similar problem in cases of myoma. How big does the myoma have to be to justify removal? They don't know.

Nonetheless, clinical conferences, tissue committees, physician education, and other strategies to eliminate unnecessary hysterectomies, plus the publicity the issue has received in both the medical literature and the lay press, may have helped a little. As I said, the hysterectomy rate *has* dropped a bit since its midseventies' peak. But these measures are not enough. The medical profession hasn't fully met its responsibilities. Again it comes down to you; you are the one who has to sign the permit to operate. If the operation has been recommended to you, ask about the benefits, the risks, the likelihood of success, and the alternatives to surgery. If you believe that indications for the operation are weak, say no. Doctor does not always know best.

9

Breast

Surgeons go about breast surgery differently now: No longer swashbucklers, taking all they can, they proceed cautiously, like diplomats, "lumpectomy" rather than the traditional "radical" mastectomy; they take small amounts, conservative as retired schoolmarms. To the surprise of many, including me, their results are just as good—or better. If their results *are* better, it's because they discover breast cancer earlier now. The big shift away from aggressive and toward limited surgery has been based on sound, controlled clinical tests of the kind that we still lack for most surgery. For breast cancer these clinical tests have clarified the limits of surgical achievement, although the picture is still not ideally clear.

Shortly after her fifty-sixth birthday, Myrna S. allowed her friend, June, to talk her into having a mammogram. First Myrna checked on the radiation dosage she would receive. "Less than a rad," said the technician she talked to on the phone. On the basis of what she had read, she decided that this amount would be all right. The mammogram was brief but slightly painful when they squeezed her breasts between two stiff plates.

Five days later her doctor called her, said a little something showed up on the X ray that should be looked into. Not much, she said, but something. After examining Myrna, her doctor said she could feel a tiny lump in the left breast, but she doubted if she would have found it except that the X ray showed exactly where it was. Myrna hadn't been able to feel it. If such a lump contained a little calcium, that would make it easier to see on X ray and would also make it quite likely to be a cancer, said the doctor, but this lump had no calcium. They couldn't tell.

The surgeon to whom Myrna was referred said he supposed they could delay. Some of these small lumps didn't change; they could X-ray it again in three months if she wanted to do that.

"No, I don't want to wait. I have to find out now. Go ahead," said Myrna. Plenty to worry about—cancer, Jesus! She could hardly sleep.

The surgeon used needles and more X rays to locate the lump precisely; then he removed the whole thing under local anesthesia—outpatient surgery. Myrna went home.

In the pathology lab thirty-six hours later, the surgeon was talking to the pathologist about the biopsy. "What do you think?"

"Here . . . you can see for yourself." The pathologist adjusted a slide under his microscope and stood up. The surgeon looked through the eyepiece. "It's fairly typical of intraductal carcinoma . . . in situ, I guess," explained the pathologist. "You can see the well-defined lobules. She doesn't have axillary nodes, does she?"

The surgeon straightened up. "No, nothing I can feel. So, I guess it's Stage I, huh? Sometimes I wonder if this kind, these little ones, are really cancer. Maybe it wouldn't grow. What do you think?"

"Well, I can't be sure about that, but it does meet our criteria for a carcinoma. I'll have to call it a carcinoma."

"Of course we'll have to go ahead," agreed the surgeon. "This is the kind we can cure . . . I think. But what about estrogen receptors? Can you test for that?"

"Yeah. We should. It might help in prognosis, but this one is too small. Not enough tissue to test."

The surgeon told Myrna that it was a tiny, early cancer and that the chances of cure were excellent (90 percent). They would excise enough of the breast, a pie-shaped segment of breast, in order to get completely around it—a segmental mastectomy—and also take out the nodes under her arm through a separate incision. After she recovered from the operation, she would have a course of x-ray therapy to the breast and the arm pit—to kill any few cancer cells that might possibly remain.

"What about chemotherapy?" She had read something about that.

"Not in your case if the nodes are negative, and I think they will be. I know it is being recommended for node-negative as well as the node-positive tumors now, but only for the ones that are bigger—two centimeters or so—not for these very small ones."

Myrna had the surgery and bore up under the x-ray treatment without complaints or complications. The lymph nodes were free of cancer, as expected. When it was all finished, her breast was only a little smaller and a little more tender than it had been before. June, her friend, said that she was proud of Myrna, and Myrna felt a little proud of herself too, but by no means relieved. Having read that one cancer makes a second one more likely, she now had to think about her next scheduled mammogram and what it might show.

FREQUENCY

Cancer of the breast is the most common malignant neoplasm and the leading cause of cancer death in women. It is the principal cause of death due to any cause in women between ages forty and forty-four (Wilson, 1986; Council on Scientific Affairs, 1984). During a lifetime, it will occur in 9 percent of females. Over 140,000 new cases appear each year, and 40,000 individuals die of it. The incidence of diagnosed breast cancer showed an 18 percent increase between 1935 and 1965 and a 50 percent increase between 1965 and 1976; however, the mortality has remained unchanged during the last forty years (Fox, 1979). The disease is less common among Japanese women and more common among infertile women and those who have their first pregnancy late in life. About 1 percent of breast cancer occurs in males.

HISTORY

Illustrations survive depicting amputation of the breast as early as 1655 (no anesthesia and only cautery to control the bleeding), and a few long-term survivals of breast amputation were reported in the eighteenth and early nineteenth centuries, but intense efforts to cure cancer of the breast surgically had to await asepsis and anesthesia. Then a burst of late nineteenth century surgical effort culminated with William Stewart Halsted's radical mastectomy in 1894 (Wangensteen, 1978).

For eighty years surgeons accepted this operation as the standard treatment for breast cancer. Based on simple concepts of cancer growth and surgical possibility, the operation made sense. Cancer starts in one small spot in the breast, they believed, then it grows and spreads out from its site of origin, first by the way of lymphatic channels to the lymph nodes in the axilla, and finally by way of the bloodstream to distant parts of the body. The surgeon could not identify the extent of spread precisely at the operating table, but if the disease had apparently not spread distantly, he could operate to remove the local disease as completely as possible and the tumor's first invasion zone, the axillary lymph nodes.

The radical mastectomy achieved those objectives. It removed all of the breast, the adjacent tissues into which the tumor might have spread, including muscles of the anterior chest wall, and the lymph nodes of the axilla. As surgeons learned to do this operation, the operative risk fell, and they attained a high cure rate when the disease was limited to the breast. When the disease had spread to the lymph nodes, however, the cure rate fell drastically.

How could they improve it? Radiation therapy was added with uncertain benefit at the time. So, several surgeons, convinced that surgery was the only hope, extended the range of the operation. They knew that the cancer spread not only to the axillary lymph nodes, which were removed during a radical mastectomy, but also to lymph nodes above the collar bone, and to nodes behind the breastbone, inside the chest. Emboldened by surgery's new technical competence, they went after these nodes and found that they could remove them in addition to the radical mastectomy with acceptable operative risk. I played a minor role in devising what we called then a "superradical mastectomy." The already considerable deformity of the radical operation was very little worse with this operation; thus if it cured significantly more patients, it would be worth the risk. Unfortunately, the results were no better than with the radical operation; the superradical operation has been abandoned.

At the same time a few dissenters, among whom should be mentioned R. McWhirter, of Scotland (1948), and George Crile, Jr., of Cleveland (1961), maintained that less aggressive surgery than the radical operation would do as well. For relatively early disease, they removed only the breast or perhaps only the tumor and then added postoperative x-ray therapy to clean up bits and pieces of tumor that might have been left or spilled during surgery. If the disease had spread beyond the breast, it wasn't apt to be cured by surgery anyway, so an aggressive surgical attack on the chest-wall muscles and the lymph nodes didn't make much sense to them. This modest estimate of surgery's possible contribution finally won out.

Controlled clinical tests conducted by the National Surgical Adjuvant Breast Project (NSABP), directed by B. Fisher of Pittsburgh (1985), showed, first, that total mastectomy or modified radical mastectomy (just the breast and the axillary nodes, not the chest-wall muscles) was as good as the radical mastectomy. As an important allied benefit, these clinical tests by the NSABP became a model of how to go about evaluating cancer treatment. In a later study, NSABP showed that segmental mastectomy for small tumors (Stage I and II), which removed only sufficient tissue to be sure that the margins of the specimen were free of tumor, followed by irradiation and by chemotherapy in women with positive nodes, was as good as total mastectomy for early disease. These lesser operations may bring about no more cures than radical mastectomy once did, but they produce much less deformity. Thus, the results of these studies have eliminated a type of excessive, if not unnecessary, surgery.

The overall improvement in treating breast cancer noted in recent years is not brought about by smaller operations or even by the addition of radiation and chemotherapy, but rather by the fact that more small tumors are being discovered and treated. Early detection rather than more effective treatment takes most of the credit. If your tumor is Stage I or II (see below for an explanation of stages), chances of cure are good, and you no longer have to have your entire breast removed—a lesson of recent surgical history.

NATURAL HISTORY OF THE DISEASE

The means to prevent breast cancer are not yet at hand, but a lot of data are. Breast cancer almost never occurs before age twenty-five, and 80 percent of it occurs in women older than forty. Heredity plays a part: The incidence is greater in women whose mothers and sisters have had breast cancer. If you've had it once, you're more apt to have it again.

The greater the number of axillary nodes invaded, the poorer the long-term survival. Breast cancer invades the lymphatics or the venous circulation or both, and about half of all patients have some spread to the axillary lymph nodes when the disease is first diagnosed. Among patients with early cancer, however, identified by mammography-screening programs, this percentage falls to 20 percent.

Classified according to its size and spread, the tumor is staged. Stage I: Less then 2 centimeters with negative nodes. Stage II: Two to 5 centimeters, negative nodes or minimally involved nodes. Stage III: Greater than 5 centimeters, positive nodes. Stage IV: Distant spread. Many of the Stage I lesions are detected only by mammography (as in Myrna's case).

The new surgical treatment I have described has come about, in part, from changes in the way we now understand the natural history of the disease. Two or more types of the disease may exist, says Maurice Fox of the Massachusetts Institute of Technology (1979). He contends that about forty percent of women afflicted finally suffer a fatal outcome relatively unaffected by treatment. In them the disease is widely distributed when first encountered clinically. The remaining 60 percent have a disease defined as cancer under the microscope, but their disease is biologically relatively benign. More patients with this latter type are discovered by modern mammography-screening techniques, and most of them would probably survive a long time no matter what the treatment. This view of the disease plays down the specific operation to which you may be subjected. Outcome depends more upon the nature of the disease than upon the nature of the treatment. If your lump is small, it's apt to have a benign, curable nature.

Disease variability is also seen in the way the tumor may or may not take up the hormones, estrogen, and progesterone (estrogen-receptor proteins). This property, measured by tests on the operative specimen, helps in predicting final outcome and in deciding what kind of treatment to use if the cancer does spread. Tumors that take up the hormones (estrogen-receptor positive) have a better prognosis and respond better to hormonal treatment (for which see below).

DIAGNOSIS

Women themselves discover most breast lumps, 80 percent of which are noncancerous, fortunately. If your doctor tells you that you need a breast biopsy for diagnosis, but that he thinks the lump is benign, he may be telling you what he really thinks. At age twenty to thirty, 1 percent of lumps are cancers, 35 percent are chronic cystic mastitis (a benign, troublesome inflammation), 30 percent are fibrous tumors, and the remaining miscellaneous lumps are also benign. Between thirty and sixty, 35 percent are mastitis and 35 percent are cancer. Over seventy years, 90 percent of lumps are cancer (Eiseman, 1980).

Because it can detect tumors that your doctor can't feel, mammography, the x-ray examination that revealed Myrna's tumor, provides the most effective way to detect small cancers. But the breast is irradiated, and radiation itself can cause cancer. When to recommend mammography requires a cost–benefit analysis that measures the cost of causing a later cancer against the benefit of detecting a present cancer early. This analysis can be a little tricky, even unconvincing. Nonetheless, with modern equipment designed solely for mammography, the x-ray dose is low.

For asymptomatic women, this is now recommended: a baseline mammogram before age forty, screening mammograms every two years from forty through forty-nine, and annual mammograms after age fifty (Council on Scientific Affairs, 1984). This schedule will pick up small tumors, but as I mentioned earlier, maybe some of these small, apparent cancers aren't really cancer—aren't, that is, invasive, lethal cancer. Unsettled issues, questions not easy to answer. In the meantime, common sense favors the periodic mammogram, although I fear its widespread use may speed our plunge into a spreading and apparently inevitable national hypochondria.

How much good does screening accomplish? Sometimes health-care proposals seem to take on the extravagant tone of advertising campaigns. If a small, curable cancer has been detected in your breast, however, screening may have done you a great deal of good. On the other hand, for those not afflicted, and therefore merely under risk, the possible general benefits of energetic cancer-detection campaigns may seem unimpressive. For example, using a mathematical model and insurance-plan data, one authority has estimated that if breast cancer were entirely eliminated, the average fifty-year-old woman, who now has a 6 percent chance of developing breast cancer, would have her life expectancy extended by only 140 days (Kunz, 1979). With the eventually fragile nature of our lives, reducing one risk seems only to open the opportunity for others.

Should you skip mammography and depend on breast self-examination instead? The National Cancer Institute of the NIH advocates breast self-examination, and provides an instructional pamphlet, but critics say that "many questions require examination" before breast self-examination can be advocated as a screening test (O'Mailey and Fletcher, 1987). Though 90 percent to 99 percent of women are aware of breast self-examination, only about 15 percent to 40 percent have actually performed it monthly.

Neither the mammogram nor the physical exam makes the definitive diagnosis. The pathologist does—on a biopsy. General or local anesthesia for the biopsy? Needle or knife? Surgeons have several options: If the lump is very tiny, X rays may be required during the biopsy in order to locate it precisely. Because of economic and psychological advantages over hospitalization, ambulatory biopsy is favored now, with a delay of several days between the biopsy and further surgery, should further surgery become necessary. As a cyst vanishes when aspirated (drawn off by suction), needle aspiration alone will settle the matter, and many benign lumps are totally removed at the time of biopsy.

A pathologist, whom you don't even get to see, peers through his microscope and makes the crucial diagnostic decision: *benign* or *malignant*. In most cases, pathologists would agree on the diagnosis of a specific specimen, if a number of them were asked to look at it. But not always. During a conference on screening methods for breast cancer a few years ago, one committee caused a stir when it reported that, as one result of a screening program, fifty-eight women had apparently had mastectomies for small nodules judged malignant that appeared to be benign on further pathology review (Kunz, 1977). The committee chairman pointed out that pathology is an "interpretive science," and that small carcinomas do cause problems.

Special problems are caused by something called "carcinoma in situ" (preinvasive) or "intraductal carcinoma" (Schnitt et al., 1988). Once considered relatively rare, carcinoma in situ is found as a small lesion (often less than 1 centimeter across) in 15 percent to 20 percent of patients undergoing mammography screening. Many of these may not really be invasive cancers at all. As the authors state: "The information available [on the risk of carcinoma in situ progressing to invasive cancer] is extremely limited." If you are tagged with one of these, you may not really have cancer, but the pathologist can't be sure. What to do? Formerly carcinoma in situ was treated with mastectomy, but today the mode is breast-conserving surgery—lumpectomy, segmental mastectomy— perhaps with radiation.

In doubtful cases pathologists consult one another but they tend to lean toward malignancy just to protect themselves. If someone comes back, after months or years, with an obvious, recurrent cancer that a pathologist had originally labeled "benign," the ax would fall. Malpractice!

Once the diagnosis "cancer," or something less decisive such as "the possibility of cancer cannot be ruled out," has been made, all clinical decisions stem from that diagnosis. The surgeon cannot disagree. He knows, of course, as does the pathologist, that certain criteria of malignancy—spreading and death if untreated—have no diagnostic utility. Your doctors have to make the best guess they can with the biopsy specimen they have. I think they do very well, but you are not in the hands of precise scientists: Medicine, we should remind ourselves, was described first as an "art"—sometime later as a "science."

THE OPERATION

I've heard surgeons describe the breast as "just a glob of fat." Though it may be beautifully formed to excite their lust and aesthetic appreciation as strongly as it does any man's, to a surgeon, as surgeon, the breast doesn't present the technical challenge of a lung or a stomach. Oh, there are the lymph nodes, a big vein at the upper part, and a couple of nerves to watch out for, but it's mostly just the problem of resecting some fat. The surgeon can easily remove a lot or a little of it, and as I said, for eighty years or so, he removed a lot. Don't worry about deformity, he told his patients; you can wear a prosthesis. He was after a cure.

Now the Halsted radical mastectomy, which removed the entire breast, much skin, two muscles of the chest wall, and the axillary lymph nodes, all in a piece, to be followed sometimes with a skin graft, has been abandoned unless a large, invasive tumor requires it.

The modified radical mastectomy (also called total mastectomy) replaced it for Stages I and II diseases—less deforming, same results. In that operation, the surgeon removes the entire breast and the lymph nodes, though not quite as completely, but he leaves the large muscles (pectoralis muscles) of the chest wall. This operation is now being replaced by even less extensive surgery.

If the tumor is quite small, your surgeon may resect only the tumor and some normal tissue beyond the tumor's margins (segmental mastectomy or lumpectomy). If he finds on pathology examination that the segmental mastectomy did not extend adequately beyond the tumor, he will sometimes at a second stage do a total mastectomy. To the segmental mastectomy he adds a separate incision through which he removes the axillary lymph nodes. There is some debate as to whether this lymph node removal is therapeutic, but it is at least informative. It allows the surgeon to classify—to stage the disease (see above).

A treatment regimen for Stages I and II tumors based on the results of a NSABP randomized clinical trial (Fisher, 1985) prescribed chemotherapy after surgery (designated, adjuvant chemotherapy) for node-positive Stage II cases but not for node-negative cases—and a course of radiation therapy for all cases. Four more recent reports extend adjuvant chemotherapy to node-negatives cases (Relman, 1989). All of these studies found that chemotherapy, and in some cases tamoxifen (an antiestrogen drug), provided small improvements in disease-free survival, but as yet no evidence of improved overall survival. These trials furnish no data on small tumors less than 2 centimeters in diameter, so chemotherapy may not be justified for them. It is certain to be used more often for other node-negative cases, however. Still lacking absolute guidelines in this changing field, you and your physician will have to keep up with new evidence as it comes in.

Your surgeon may, in good conscience, not want to adhere to all features of these regimens. He is, I would think, most likely (particularly if he was trained to do radical mastectomies) to object to the lumpectomy and recommend a total mastectomy instead. "There may be other small, hidden cancers in the same breast," he might say, or, "I'm not sure I can get around it," or "Not all the evidence is in." But you should keep in mind that the best current evidence, based on controlled clinical tests, does favor the less deforming operation for small, that is for Stages I and II, cancers.

Breast preservation or restoration has gone beyond the use of these partial mastectomies. Surgeons now insert about 100,000 silicone breast implants a year, and many women ask for augmentation mammoplasty following a mastectomy (Goldwyn, 1987). If your operation is a segmental mastectomy, you may not need to consider it, but it could enhance your nude appearance after a total mastectomy. In one sense this is unnecessary surgery: Obviously the operation does nothing to improve your chances of survival. It could even harm your chances. I wonder if a surgeon, planning for a later augmentation mammoplasty, might not, unpremeditated, take out less tissue then he should at the original resection in order to make his later, plastic-reconstruction operation easier. To me it's a plausible fault. I believe I used to compromise my skin excision for a radical mastectomy in order to avoid the fuss of a skin graft.

Many women find that the idea of having an augmentation mammoplasty helps their self-esteem. If your doctor recommends it, or you decide to look into it, keep in mind that although it can be done immediately (Feller, 1986), it usually requires from one to three additional operations, it's expensive, and silicone, because it becomes stiff, is a poor substitute for flesh. If you get a chance, feel someone's reconstructed breast yourself.

Although wound complications do occur in about 10 percent of cases, the mortality of breast surgery is low—less then 1 in 1,000.

RESULTS

Results are reported as survival rather than as cure, because occasionally the disease will recur late, to wipe out a "cure," twenty years or more after surgery. The most important predictor of survival is the state of the axillary lymph nodes at the time of surgery. Negative nodes: five-year survival of 78 percent; ten-year survival of 50 percent. Positive nodes: five-year survival of 50 percent; ten-year survival of 33 percent. If the disease has spread to the chest wall and skin before surgery: five-year survival of 20 percent; ten-year survival of 10 percent (Eiseman, 1980). Although survival for a specific stage of the disease has not changed over the years, overall survival has improved because more node-negative tumors are discovered and treated. This and the long useful life possible even without cure are the best news about the disease.

Other predictors of outcome are the estrogen-receptor level of the tumor, the growth-doubling time of the tumor cells, and the DNA content (diploid or aneuploid). The latter may turn out to be the most accurate prognosticator.

SPECIAL PROBLEMS, ADVANCED BREAST CANCER

Breast cancer appearing during pregnancy or lactation tends to grow faster than usual. During the first half of pregnancy, it is treated with mastectomy but without radiation, because of potential fetal damage. If it appears during the second half of pregnancy, treatment may be delayed until after delivery or the pregnancy interrupted. Cancers arising during lactation are treated conventionally after suppressing lactation (Wilson, 1986).

Each year approximately 1 percent of patients who have had breast cancer manifest the disease in the opposite breast (five times the usual rate). Concern about this high incidence has led to the recommendation of a blind biopsy of the opposite breast at the time of mastectomy—rarely done, I would think—but an annual mammogram of the remaining breast (or of both breasts if the mastectomy was partial) makes sense.

One to 2 percent of breast cancer occurs in males, where it tends to spread early and have a poor prognosis. If it can be resected with a mastectomy, however, five-year survival has been good. When recurrent or widespread, it often responds to castration, a type of hormonal therapy.

Hormonal therapy often plays an important part in the treatment of advanced female breast cancer too, as do radiation and chemotherapy, a triumvirate that achieves better relief and longer survival here than with most other advanced cancers, partly because breast cancer, by its nature, may grow slowly. Dramatic remissions (as well as distressing side effects) have resulted from each of these therapies. They are often employed one after the other, in hope of getting several remissions—the primary objective being to improve the quality rather than the length of survival.

Recurrences that require treatment usually appear within the first five years: locally (near the site of the primary disease) in 25 percent, in the bones in 25 percent, in the lungs in 20 percent, and someplace else in the remaining 30 percent. Radiation is particularly effective for local disease and for bone spread, achieving at least temporary remission in 90 percent of local disease and a relief of bone pain caused by metastases in 75 percent of cases.

Combination chemotherapy (several chemicals at once) has been more effective than a single chemotherapeutic agent, achieving some response in about 75 percent of cases, for a median duration of about nine months.

As hormonal therapy may involve surgical removal of endocrine glands and the administration of powerful drugs, it has become complex enough to confuse all but an expert and toxic enough to cause debilitating and dangerous side effects. Nonetheless, it may significantly prolong useful life. Male hormones, female hormones (estrogen), corticosteroids, and antifemale-sex-hormone drugs may be used. Whether the patient is pre- or postmenopausal becomes important; there is no point in using estrogen (the female hormone) premenopausally, but it has produced remission in about 36 percent of postmenopausal women. Though androgen, the male hormone, has many undesirable side effects, including interconversion to estrogen (unwanted for these patients), it brings about remissions in about 20 percent of either pre- or postmenopausal women. Corticosteroids cause fewer side effects than androgen, and they are credited with remissions in about half the cases. An antiestrogen drug, tamoxifen (also used with adjuvant chemotherapy during primary treatment—see above), causes remission in about 40 percent of cases.

First advocated in 1896, oophorectomy (removing the ovaries) was for many years the only hormone-related operation for breast cancer patients. A controlled study many years ago has shown that it did not help when done at the time of the primary mastectomy, but it is often the initial therapeutic trial in premenopausal women with recurrent breast cancer. Or, alternatively, the ovarian function may be suppressed with radiation to avoid surgery, though with radiation the effect is slower.

In postmenopausal women or after an initial success with oophorectomy followed by recurrence, adrenalectomy (removing hormone glands near the kidneys) or hypophysectomy (removing the pituitary, a hormone master gland at the base of the brain) may be tried. Since it is a less formidable operation that achieves similar results, most therapists, other than neurosurgeons, prefer adrenalectomy. After either of these operations, replacement hormone administration will require continuing care.

The problem of deciding which of these various therapies to use for advanced cancer has provoked a lot of high-class research (estrogen-receptor investigation, which I mentioned earlier, is an example); much of this has paid off in better understanding of the disease and in palliation. But since these techniques and treatments don't cure advanced disease, they are examples, once again, of the halfway technology we have encountered in other fields of modern medicine while we wait for definitive treatment.

ALTERNATIVES

Chemotherapy, hormonal therapy, and radiation, as I have described their use, are not alternative treatments. Rather, they are treatments supplemental to, or parallel with surgery, whose effectiveness has been quite well defined by controlled studies. Modern treatment of breast cancer has become multimodal and often, it seems, unremitting.

Presently, radiotherapy as primary treatment offers the only rational alternative to mastectomy (Moxley, 1980). Trials are in progress both in the United States and Europe. Reports that have been made tell of local control as good as that achieved with surgery, but no long-term survival comparisons have been reported yet. Better breast preservation than that achieved by a segmental mastectomy would be the principle benefit; the disadvantage would be the general debility, long treatment period, and possible unrelated damage caused by heavy radiation.

I'll comment on unproved and unscientific alternative treatments in Chapter 16. The same alternatives that are used for many other cancers tend to be used for breast cancer. They include such things as laetrile, krebiozen, the Simonton approach, high-dose vitamin C, homeopathy, and a fascinating array of less well-known nostrums.

10

Gallbladder

After inspecting the ultrasound pictures of his patient's gallbladder, a surgeon friend of mine, now in his midsixties, said, "I've ordered this on a lot of patients, but I've never actually seen how the thing works."

"Let me show you," volunteered the ultrasonographer. "Nothing to it. Of course you know there's no radiation and no special preparation. It only takes a couple of minutes. Here, climb up on the table—for free, in your case—let's get your belt out of the way." He helped the surgeon climb on to the examination table. "I'll do your gallbladder. As you know, it's really good for that."

Right, took only a few minutes, no pain, no radiation—but what did they find? Gallstones! The ultrasound image showed gallstones. Who wants that? When my surgeon friend was telling me about this later, he used the fingers of both hands to press into his abdomen, just below the ribs on the right, as if he were trying to feel the damn stones he now knew were undeniably there. Did he find a tender spot when he pressed? "One of those stones is about a centimeter in diameter," he said. He had seen it, and there were probably some small ones that might work their way down into the ducts and cause real trouble later on.

"Jesus!" I said, "you're not going to have a cholecystectomy are you? Everyone over sixty—or at least a lot of us over sixty—has gallstones. Why did you let him take that stupid picture in the first place?"

My friend gestured helplessly. The deed had been done. Now he had to live with the stones or undergo major surgery. He was in a position common to clients who have too many regular checkups: The SOBs always manage to find something.

He still hasn't had the operation, but who knows? Many persons, including surgeons who should know better, have cholecystectomies for indications no more compelling than his.

Critics who write about unnecessary surgery may not even list chole-cystectomy as unnecessary, yet many of these operations *are* unnecessary. For years otherwise competent and conscientious surgeons have been recommending cholecystectomy for silent gallstones (cause no symptoms—the kind my surgeon friend has) (Glen, 1983). If they discover the stones incidentally—say, on an X ray taken for some other reason— these surgeons recommend surgery. Thereby, they say, you can avoid trouble later on. Fine, nice to avoid trouble later on, but most silent stones remain silent. Autopsy examinations have shown that about 30 percent of persons over age sixty have gallstones (Eiseman, 1980), most of which have never caused any trouble.

It's hard to criticize a surgeon who takes out a gallbladder (operation is called cholecystectomy) full of stones; he has the evidence of genuine disease right there rattling in his specimen tray. The tissue committee, which I have mentioned in Chapter 8, won't complain. They are looking for real pathology, and this is real pathology. Not like a normal uterus, the extirpation of which may demand from the surgeon some sort of a mealymouthed explanation. Stones are abnormal. But should they always be surgically removed?

FREQUENCY

Surgeons have been busily doing just that for a long time. In 1986 they removed 502,000 gallbladders in the United States, making cholecystec-tomy the second most frequent general surgical operation—outranked only by hernia repair. Decidedly a lot of surgery, but there are a lot of general surgeons, each of whom wants abundant surgery. The number of general surgeons increased by 13 percent between 1979 and 1984, but the number of general surgical operations increased by only 7 percent, leaving fewer operations per surgeon (Rutkow, 1986). They have lost the chest to thoracic surgeons, the head and neck to ear-nose-and-throat surgeons, and the large bowel to proctologists. Left with gallbladders, hernias, varicose veins, and sundry items, general surgeons require all they can legitimately procure. Hospitals, too, need a dependable source of gall-bladder clients from which to fill their pockets. Don't you become a partial solution to their plight. Unless you find a clear need to dispose of it, keep your gallbladder.

HISTORY

Gallstones, no recent disease of industrial civilization and modern stress, have been discovered in mummies of the 21st Egyptian dynasty, but they weren't assaulted surgically until the nineteenth century A.D. The first cholecystectomy (1882, in Berlin) was followed in 1886 by the first American cholecystectomy (Nahrwold, 1986). Made possible with asepsis and general anesthesia, and made accurate with diagnostic techniques that became available in the twentieth century, the operation has fared well. But doctors still haven't figured out, with convincing evidence, precisely when it is really needed.

NATURAL HISTORY OF THE DISEASE

The gallbladder is a storage sack, slightly larger than a thumb, attached to the undersurface of the liver on the right side, and connected by its duct (the cystic duct) to a larger duct (the common bile duct) that runs from the liver to the first part of the intestine (the duodenum). A digestive juice (bile), manufactured by the liver, passes through the common bile duct to the duodenum where it mixes with the food. But when digestion stops, the opening of the common duct into the duodenum closes, and bile, still secreted by the liver, backs up into the gallbladder. Then when bile is needed again, the common duct opens and the gallbladder evacuates its stored bile.

If, for reasons not fully understood, the concentrations of stored chemicals in the bile become too great for the amount of solvent, saturation occurs, and crystals may form, which become the nuclei of gradually developing stones in the relatively stagnant gallbladder pool. Three kinds of stones may form: cholesterol (same substance that causes trouble in the arteries) stones, pigment stones, or mixed stones. The formation process produces chronic cholecystitis with inflammation and thickening of the gallbladder wall.

If a small stone plugs the gallbladder duct, suddenly preventing evacuation, the resulting painful gallbladder distention, acute cholecystitis, may, in the worst case, progress to gangrene of the gallbladder. The obstruction due to a stone may, however, develop slowly, producing an enormous gallbladder known as hydrops of the gallbladder. Or the gallbladder may become inflamed, to produce acute cholecystitis, in debilitated patients without either obstruction of its duct or stones.

If stones pass into the common bile duct, they may plug that duct, causing a liver backup and jaundice. Sometimes stones that have passed into the common bile duct may obstruct the pancreatic duct (a duct that enters the duodenum with the common duct) and cause inflammation of the pancreas (pancreatitis).

Women of childbearing age have a higher incidence of gallbladder disease than men of the same age, and the old have more trouble than the young. As I said, 30 percent of people over sixty have stones. Cirrhosis predisposes to pigment stones as do blood diseases that cause destruction of red cells. Cancer of the gallbladder does occur with gallstones but infrequently, less than 1 percent.

DIAGNOSIS

Recurrent short bouts of sharp pain in the right upper region of the abdomen, usually following meals, sometimes relieved by vomiting, may be "biliary colic" that can be attributed to gallstones. If the acute attack becomes steady, instead of colicky, with fever and conspicuous tenderness in the right upper abdomen, this too may be due to the gallbladder as an attack of "acute cholecystitis." In either case, if this is your story, your doctor will probably blame your symptoms on your gallbladder, particularly if he finds stones on ultrasonography.

Experience suggests that in these cases he's right: The gallbladder caused the symptoms. Other symptoms, without the colicky pain, are often blamed on the gallbladder but offer unconvincing evidence of gallbladder disease. Intolerance to fatty foods, flatulence, bloating, belching, heartburn, and other vague digestive symptoms are often charged to the gallbladder just because stones are present. The relationship may be coincidental. Vague digestive complaints may be due to peptic ulcer, inflammation of the stomach lining (gastritis), constipation, anxiety, nervousness, coronary heart disease, psychoneurosis, and so forth. The doctor may too quickly blame the stones, because he finds it impossible, or excessively time-consuming, to assign them more certainly to one or more of these other, often vague, causes. He has to make a definitive diagnosis quickly; his patient expects him to. A confession of medical ignorance, often the correct alternative, may be intolerable to both patient and doctor.

Although the uncertainty of trying to connect symptoms to gallstones can be disconcerting, the excellent techniques for diagnosing the presence of stones are reassuring. Today, the diagnosis of gallstones is usually confirmed by ultrasound examination, a sensitive, highly accurate technique that uses no radiation or dyes, as did earlier diagnostic methods. Stones in the common duct, a special problem, are identified by endoscopy or by techniques for injecting dye directly into that deeply concealed duct before X rays are taken. Occasionally a CAT (computer assisted tomography) scan may be used. Some diagnosticians say that they can't absolutely exclude coronary artery disease, in questionable cases, as a cause of upper abdominal pain unless the coronary arteries themselves are viewed by coronary angiogram, but the much simpler electrocardiography may resolve this diagnostic puzzle.

INDICATIONS

Acute cholecystitis, a good reason for recommending cholecystectomy, may be treated nonsurgically, but then the course of the disease is drawn out, and cholecystectomy is, in any case, finally required. Perhaps as many as 20 percent of cholecystectomies are done for acute cholecystitis. If that has been the indication for your surgery, this chapter obviously will not have helped you make your decision, but for other indications it may guide you.

Other good reasons for recommending surgery are recurrent attacks of the biliary colic I have described above. So are stones in the common duct that cause obstruction and jaundice.

In contrast, vague abdominal complaints and asymptomatic gallstones are poor indications. The mortality rate for cholecystectomy is 0.3 percent, usually considered an acceptable risk. But George Crile, Jr. (1978), pointed out that if, as a conservative estimate, say, 10 million people in the United States have asymptomatic gallstones, and all of these people submitted to a cholecystectomy (a real bonanza for surgeons!), 30,000 people would die unnecessarily. If through some kind of a workup or checkup a doctor finds your asymptomatic gallstones and recommends an operation, say *no*. As with my friend the surgeon, you would have been better off not to have had the checkup in the first place. In any case, forget the stones—if you can.

Your doctor may recommend the operation if you have complained of heartburn, "dyspepsia," or indigestion, and during his workup he finds gallstones on ultrasound. After surgery done for these indications, many patients complain less of their indigestion, at least for a while. But the gallstones may not have caused the symptoms, or the operation the cure. People without stones also complain of dyspepsia and indigestion, and improve with time or with nonsurgical treatments. The stones may have been incidental rather than causal, and the powerful placebo effect of surgery may have elicited the improvement.

THE OPERATION

The surgeon operates through an abdominal incision made parallel to the margin of the ribs on the right, or through an up-and-down incision near the midline. The gallbladder, accessible just under the margin of the liver on the right, is detached from the bottom up or from the top down, and its duct is tied off where it joins the common duct. Abnormal anatomy and stones in the common duct provoke the major surgical problems. If he can't identify the problem correctly, the surgeon may injure or divide the common duct—a serious, chronic, sometimes fatal complication. If stones are present in the common duct, the surgeon should remove them, but he may not find them. His search for them is aided by X rays of the common duct during surgery.

In large series, the risk of death from the surgery has been about 0.5 percent, falling to 0.1 percent among those under age fifty, and rising to 2 percent in those over seventy. The most frequent cause of death is heart or vascular disease with liver disease, such as cirrhosis, next (Nahrwold, 1986).

RESULTS

After cholecystectomy, most patients no longer complain of their preoperative symptoms, but when they do complain, surgeons call this unfortunate event the postcholecystectomy syndrome, and attribute it to having left the stump of the gallbladder duct too long, or to other nonsense such as something called biliary dyskinesia. As a matter of fact, the patient probably still has the same, ill-defined, inaccurately diagnosed, possibly psychoneurotic indigestion that he started out with. His problem may never be fully understood. Clinical medicine is embarrassed by many commonplace uncertainties such as this, and no early solutions are likely.

ALTERNATIVES

Progress in the gallstone market has taken the form of still largely experimental techniques to dissolve the stones with chemicals or to break them up with shock waves. Because these methods may save you from surgery, they will be welcome, but if they are to be employed in a campaign to rid those 10 million, or more, quiet gallbladders of their silent stones, I will object. We could have an epidemic of unnecessary lithotripsy instead of unnecessary cholecystectomy.

Shock wave lithotripsy has worked successfully to break up kidney stones, and the same technique has now been applied experimentally to gallstones (Sackmann et al., 1988). Carefully selected patients with one to three gallstones have been subjected to focused, high-energy shock waves usually under general anesthesia and while immersed in a water bath. The stones are reduced to a sludge that is expected to pass out of the gall-bladder if assisted by adjuvant medical therapy. At present, the technique is almost as complex as an operation—not yet ready for general clinical application.

In some patients, predominantly cholesterol gallstones can be dissolved by the oral administration of chenodeoxycholic acid. Because of various reasons, however, such as the presence of large stones or a nonfunctioning gallbladder, most patients are unsuitable for this treatment. In a recent Swedish study, only twenty-two patients out of 342 turned out to be suitable (Welch and Malt, 1987). Twelve of these were treated, and one had dissolution of the stones.

Perhaps methyl tert-butyl ether (MTBE) will turn out to be more practical. This, too, is used to dissolve cholesterol stones, but it must be injected directly into the gallbladder through a catheter rather than taken orally. The Mayo clinic has reported its use in seventy-five patients with cholesterol gallstones, in whom there was complete dissolution or more than 95 percent dissolution of stones in seventy-two (Thistle et al., 1989). Hospitalization is required, and some have had recurrence, but they conclude that MTBE is a useful alternative to surgery.

Your best alternative to cholecystectomy now may be simply to forget about the stones if they are silent; no need to have this part of your internal anatomy redone surgically. If you think the stones are causing symptoms, you might avoid fatty foods and lose some weight. The modern, prudent, low-fat diet for vigorous Americans advocated by the American Heart Association (for other reasons, of course), by other prestigious committees, and by countless individual nutritionists and diet-book writers may do the trick.

11

Appendectomy

Emergency surgery—recommended by your doctor while your belly aches, and you cower in an emergency room—hardly provides time to look it up in this book. Before you reached that emergency room, however, you should have made important decisions: to seek help and where to go first—to a family practitioner, to an emergency room, or to a surgeon. In Chapter 20 I deal with the choice of a surgeon—information that might have helped you face the emergency. If you now want to learn about appendicitis, this chapter will help you too, for it describes what goes on during the process of the disease, what physicians have learned about appendicitis and how they learned. Appendicitis is still a common disease—with a most interesting history.

The modern surgical treatment of appendicitis has worked to reduce the death rate of the disease from 15 per 100,000 per year in 1930 to 0.7 recently. In 1935 appendicitis ranked fifteenth among causes of death in the United States, accounting for 16,000 deaths; by 1973, with a greatly increased population, it caused only 1,000 deaths (Wangensteen, 1978). A decreased incidence of the disease—cause unknown—accounts for much of this improvement, but an aggressive surgical program also deserves credit: Operate at the beginning of the disease, before perforation, when there may still be some doubt about the diagnosis. As might be expected, the surgeon who follows this program ends up with not a few normal appendices in his specimen pan (about 20 percent), but the 80 percent with appendicitis will have avoided the dread progression to perforation and peritonitis (Preston, 1983). A surgical textbook states the accepted principle (Condon, 1986): "The only way to reduce morbidity and to prevent mortality is to perform appendectomy before perforation or gangrene has occurred."

The individual who, submitting to this program, has had his normal appendix removed may then wonder: Was this, too, an "unnecessary" operation? I have described many unnecessary operations in this book, but for suspected appendicitis, managed prudently in fitting circumstances, the removal of a normal appendix is unavoidable rather than unnecessary. The risk has been low, and the population undergoing appendectomy, as a whole, has benefited from the aggressive program. If this seems like a turnabout from my warnings about unnecessary coronary bypasses, hysterectomies, cholecystectomies, cesarean sections, tonsillectomies—also examples of surgery practiced aggressively—remember that appendicitis often follows a rapid, potentially fatal course. The diseases for which these other operations are done can be treated unhurriedly and nonsurgically, as well as, or better than, with surgery.

A thirty-one-year-old actor, who for a couple of months had been taking bicarbonate of soda for his indigestion, had an attack of abdominal pain, severe enough by Monday morning to bring him to a New York hospital. Here at six o'clock that same evening he had an appendectomy that took about an hour (Mackenzie, 1974). Three hours later he awoke from the anesthesia and seemed all right, but by the next morning his doctors discovered that peritonitis had developed. Despite this grave complication, the actor appeared to improve a little over the next few days. Many in attendance, however, expressed concern.

Crowds of his fans tried to invade the hospital; cables and telegrams poured in from all over the world. This actor was none other than the matchless Rudolph Valentino!

By Saturday his condition had deteriorated. Four physicians who were summoned agreed that things had taken a turn for the worse. Still another physician was called, but to no avail—wise, gray heads mumbled inconsequentially. The mass gathering outside the hospital became, with growing, bitter certainty, a death watch. Valentino died a week after surgery, on August 23, 1926.

Headlines in an extra edition of the *Washington Times* reported the death in type as large as had been used for the death of President Harding. In front of the hospital, a mass demonstration of feminine grief and hysteria injured many mourners. One of Valentino's physicians suffered a heart attack and was hospitalized himself. Rumors swept Broadway that Valentino had been murdered by poisoning (some jealous male?), but his surgeon announced that the "cause of death was sepsis." No autopsy was done.

Valentino's case ends as a mystery with an incomplete diagnosis, but a common opinion among surgeons has been that the actor really had a perforated peptic ulcer rather than appendicitis. When the appendix is removed in such cases, it may show superficial inflammation, as would all surfaces within the abdomen after a perforation, and thus suggest an erroneous diagnosis of appendicitis. Unless the surgeon recognizes the trouble at the operating table and promptly makes a second incision to reach and repair the perforation, peritonitis will advance to cause the "sepsis" that killed Valentino.

This same diagnostic confusion may occur today. Though in most cases appendicitis follows a predictable course, accurate preoperative diagnosis may elude the surgeon, who during surgery must remain flexible, prepared to change his mind and respond boldly to the evidence.

FREQUENCY

Among general surgical operations, appendectomy, at 275,000 a year, stands fourth. It's preceded by hernia repair, cholecystectomy (gallbladder removal), and lysis (freeing up) of adhesions. Lysis of adhesions, the third most common general surgical operation is, by the way, a surgically generated cause of surgery. Adhesions, you see, are a late complication of any abdominal surgery. (Refer to the case of Maria K. described in Chapter 8.)

For unknown reasons, but possibly because of the widespread use of antibiotics or a dietary change providing more roughage, the incidence of appendicitis decreased strikingly in the United States after about 1940. Despite a 15 percent increase in our population, surgeons performed 16 percent fewer appendectomies in 1968 than they did a decade earlier.

Rare in infants, the disease becomes increasingly more common throughout childhood, reaching a maximum incidence in the teens and twenties. It is the most frequent cause of persisting, progressive abdominal pain in teenagers. Among them, the male–female ration is about 3 to 2. This ratio decreases, reaching 1–1 in middle age, and the incidence falls off in old people. At present rates the risk at birth of developing appendicitis during a lifetime is about 1 in 5 for males and 1 in 6 for females.

HISTORY

Leonardo da Vinci depicted the appendix in an anatomical drawing he made in 1492, but no progress was made in recognizing or treating appendicitis, until the late nineteenth century (Williams, 1983). The frequently fatal inflammation that occurred in the right-lower abdomen had been called "typhlitis" or "perityphlitis" before Reginald Fitz, a pathologist, described appendicitis accurately in 1886 and recommended appendectomy as cure. After Fitz's paper, doctors began recognizing the disease early, and if they could remove the appendix before it perforated, they cured it. But early diagnosis was not always possible, and delay was sure to threaten even the mighty (Williams, 1983).

Edward, heir apparent to the British crown, had few serious responsibilities when he was young, but after his mother, Queen Victoria, died in 1901, Edward, at fifty-nine, became king. His coronation as Edward VII was set for June 26, 1902. Lamentably, and to the dismay of his court, twelve days before the coronation, Edward complained of a belly ache. He was seen promptly by the physician-in-ordinary to the King. By midnight Edward complained of more pain, and a consultant was called. They delayed. On the sixteenth, ten days before coronation, Edward proceeded by carriage to Windsor Castle, where he was seen by Sir Frederick Treves, a surgeon who found a swelling in the right-lower part of the abdomen and noted a fever. Fortunately these findings seemed to abate, and during the next couple of days the King recovered sufficiently to depart for London, where he hosted a large dinner party for coronation guests.

After the party Edward relapsed. At 10 A.M. the following morning the assembled royal physicians agreed that, despite the enormous inconvenience of the whole thing, surgery was necessary. But the King hesitated; he must attend the coronation on schedule. Said Sir Frederick Treves, "Then, Sir, you will go as a corpse."

On the 24th an appendicial abscess was drained under general anesthesia without removing the appendix itself. Treves stayed in attendance with the King for seven sleepless nights, and the King recovered. But to the general consternation of florists, functionaries, caterers, and many royal visitors the coronation had to be delayed until August 12.

NATURAL HISTORY OF THE DISEASE

The appendix is a pencil-sized, blind-ended tube attached to the beginning of the large intestine. It worms about purposelessly in the right-lower corner of the abdomen, waiting to cause trouble. A small, stonelike bit of stool (called a fecalith) or an overgrowth of the lymphatic tissue normally found in its wall may plug the tube's orifice. When that happens, fluid accumulates, pressure builds up behind the obstruction, the tube distends and becomes inflamed. If the process continues, the pressure in the tube may block the circulation; gangrene and perforation follow. The bacteria-laden contents escape into the normally sterile abdominal cavity, causing peritonitis, which if uncontrolled and generalized, will kill.

In typical cases this pathological scenario is accompanied by a characteristic progression of symptoms and physical findings. Symptoms begin with middle, or upper-middle, abdominal pain and a loss of appetite, followed by nausea and perhaps vomiting, and a low-grade fever. After a while, a few hours usually, the pain moves to the right side and then down to the region of the appendix in the right lower region of the abdomen. Though there are many variations of this typical story, pain is always present, until it is relieved, in some cases temporarily, by perforation.

The typical physical sign of appendicitis is local tenderness in the right lower quadrant (often at a specific point called McBurney's point). When the examining doctor presses a distant part of the abdomen and then suddenly releases his pressure, a stab of pain is felt at McBurney's point. Rectal examination and pelvic examination confirm the location of the tenderness and rule out some other diseases.

If appendicitis progresses to gangrene and perforation, the process may be contained at first in the right lower abdomen as an abscess—the case with Edward VII—or it may spread quickly throughout the abdominal cavity, causing general abdominal tenderness and rapid clinical deterioration.

Perforation occurs in about 20 percent of cases during the first twenty-four hours and in about 70 percent of cases by forty-eight hours. In infants and in children under five, the perforation rate reaches 80 percent, and in the elderly, too, the perforation rate rises. Fortunately, the disease is relatively uncommon among the very young and the very old.

Acute appendicitis may subside spontaneously to recur as chronic appendicitis—an unusual event. Appendectomy for "chronic" appendicitis is rarely justified. A previously inflamed appendix will show the scars of its inflammation, but the scars of an old appendicial inflammation usually don't cause pain.

DIAGNOSIS

In over half the cases, the experienced surgeon may diagnose appendicitis entirely on the basis of the clinical symptoms and physical signs I have described. When the picture is not quite typical for appendicitis, a more thorough diagnostic study may reach other conclusions. For example, a perforated peptic ulcer—the disease that killed Rudolph Valentino—will on X ray show free air in the spaces of the abdomen where it shouldn't be. Blood-chemistry measurements will identify inflammation of the pancreas (pancreatitis) as the cause of a pain sometimes confused with that caused by appendicitis. Red cells in the urine may mean a kidney stone. Among newer diagnostic techniques ultrasonography now appears to be a useful aid, which we are sure to see used more often (Puylaert, 1987), and computer analysis of the clinical manifestations, to reinforce or to alter the clinician's opinion, may increase diagnostic accuracy. Still, as in the past, some uncertainty will doubtless remain.

Ann T., a college junior, came to the dispensary at 5 P.M. Monday, complaining of nausea and abdominal pain. After hospital admission and examination by me, the surgeon, at 6:15 P.M., she said she felt a little better. The pain had gone away. Did she want to eat? No, but she was ready to leave and go back to the dormitory.

I found that her abdomen was a little tender on the right, but not much. On rectal and pelvic exams, I found nothing significant. Her temperature was 99.2 degrees and her white blood count normal. "You'd better stay in all night," I said. "We'll see in the morning."

Next morning her temperature was 102 degrees, and her abdomen was tender throughout. Antibiotics were started and preparations made for emergency surgery. I removed a perforated appendix, placed antibiotics in the belly. For twenty-four hours Ann had a high fever and a high pulse rate, but she recovered without wound complications and was back in school ten days following her appendectomy.

The surgical diagnostician will find a number of cases that could be appendicitis, but about which he can't be sure. If he waits, as I did, maybe the trouble, whatever it is, will subside. On the other hand, you can see what might happen. In this case, luck was on Ann's side—and mine, the miscreant. It's best to err in the other direction, in the direction of early surgery. Early surgery sacrifices diagnostic accuracy, but it saves lives. Mark Ravitch, a surgical aphorist whom I have quoted elsewhere, when advising other surgeons said, "There is only one way to have a 100 percent accurate diagnostic record for acute appendicitis, and that is to wait until they all rupture."

Some conditions likely to be confused with appendicitis can be accurately diagnosed to avoid surgery. By noting the time of last menstruation, the pain (Mittelschmerz) that sometimes occurs when the ovarian follicle bursts normally to discharge the egg, can be identified. Myocardial infarction (heart attack), pneumonia, and urinary tract infections, each of which may cause abdominal pain, and acute pancreatitis, which always causes abdominal pain, can be identified. Gastroenteritis (inflammation of the stomach and intestines), inflammation of a congenital blind pouch of the intestine (Meckel's diverticulum), inflammation of the distal small bowel (regional enteritis or Crohn's disease—Eisenhower had this, remember?), infected diverticulae of the large bowel (diverticulitis), salpingitis (infection of the Fallopian tubes), endometriosis (described in Chapter 8), ectopic pregnancy, perforated peptic ulcer (Valentino's problem), and inversion of the bowel upon itself in children (intussusception) are more difficult to distinguish from appendicitis preoperatively. They may not be identified until the abdomen is opened at surgery. This is true, too, of an enlargement of the lymph nodes that drain the small intestine (mesenteric lymphadenitis), which is a common finding when the surgeon encounters a normal appendix at surgery.

THE OPERATION

If he makes a diagnosis of "probable appendicitis" or "acute abdomen" of undetermined cause, your surgeon will recommend surgery. He'll take time to administer fluids and start prophylactic antibiotics, then, usually under general anesthesia and through a transverse incision—vertical if there is considerable diagnostic uncertainty—he'll find the cecum (the first part of the large intestine) and attached to it, as a blind-ended tube, the appendix. If the appendix is the villain, he takes it out and quits; if it was perforated, he increases the antibiotic dosage. In that case he may leave the superficial part of the wound open and close it later, a plan that helps avoid wound infection (a common complication if there has been a perforation). If the appendix is normal, he explores, searching for a cause that he may be able to remedy.

If the appendix has ruptured before surgery and produced an abscess, he may only drain the abscess (the operation that Edward VII had) or drain the abscess and remove the appendix—a matter of surgical judgment.

Another matter of surgical judgment, unrelated to an attack of acute appendicitis, is when to do an incidental appendectomy—removal of the normal appendix incidental to some other abdominal operation. Many surgeons do this—justifiably I think—when the appendix is easily accessible at the finish of an uncomplicated abdominal operation.

The mortality of acute nongangrenous appendicitis is less than 0.1 percent. It rises to about 0.6 percent in gangrenous appendicitis and approximately 5 percent in perforated appendicitis (Condon, 1986). Most of the deaths are among patients with diffuse peritonitis. Series of several hundred consecutive appendectomies have been reported with no mortality.

Complications, mostly wound infections, occur in 5 percent of unperforated cases and in 30 percent of cases with gangrene or perforation. Intra-abdominal or pelvic abscesses are fairly common, and the usual array of lung, heart, and urinary tract complications may follow—as they may follow any general surgical operation. Intestinal obstruction due to postoperative adhesions occurs late and may require surgery. The same inflammation that produces these obstruction-causing adhesions may plug the Fallopian tubes and cause tubal infertility, particularly following perforation. One report estimated that 5 percent of tubal infertility in the United States could be the result of perforated appendicitis (Mueller, 1986).

ALTERNATIVES

Some years ago H. L. Mencken, who criticized the Medical Trust as well as the quacks of his time, said of chiropractic (Mencken, 1927)—a possible alternative treatment then, perhaps even now—that, "If a man, being ill of a pus appendix, resorts to a shaved and fumigated longshoreman to have it disposed of, and submits willingly to a treatment involved balancing him on McBurney's spot and playing on his vertebrae as on a concertina, then I am willing, for one, to believe that he is badly wanted in Heaven."

Mencken's blunt irony may be too harsh for my modern readers who are tolerant of "alternative therapies," but now, as then, orthodox surgery provides the best treatment for a pus appendix.

If there is no possibility of surgery at hand, however, antibiotics can be used as an effective alternative. They are safer than unskilled surgery, but not as safe as skilled surgery. With antibiotics alone, a quarter of the appendices will go on to perforate and 5 to 10 percent of the patients will die (Eiseman, 1980).

In the usual case of appendicitis, antibiotics are started before surgery, not as definitive treatment but rather prophylactically, to reduce the likelihood of spreading infection in case a perforated appendix is found. If the appendix is intact, the antibiotics are discontinued postoperatively; if it's perforated, they are continued at increased dosage.

We don't know how to prevent appendicitis, but since its incidence has dropped in recent decades, speculation turns to the possible effects of widely prescribed antibiotics and the effects of a diet that modern marketing, modern agriculture, and nutritional enthusiasm have promoted. A high-fiber diet moves the bulkier stools faster; fecaliths don't have time to form and plug the appendix. Some investigators say that people in underdeveloped countries where diets are high in fiber don't have much appendicitis. The incidence of appendicitis increases, they say, with improved milling techniques and increased consumption of refined foods and sugar.

12

Hernia

With hernia, the problem is not unnecessary surgery as much as it is failed surgery. Most hernias ought to be repaired: The risk of surgery is low, initial success is good, but too often the hernia reappears.

F.G., a 54-year-old accountant, had lived with his inguinal (groin) hernia for about ten years. He backpacked on his vacations, jogged regularly, and sometimes pushed a little iron. When he coughed, however, he had to flex his thigh or press his fist into his groin to keep his guts in place. If he did this in company, his wife would grimace and roll her eyes. F.G. didn't consider this protective behavior especially debilitating. He had been reassured by a doctor who, after examining him prior to a long trip, told him that the hernia was "direct," it wouldn't likely "strangulate" in a foreign land. Grim sound to that word, but F.G., with perhaps a characteristic stoicism, managed not to worry—much.

Still, the thing *was* getting bigger, and now his job provided good medical coverage. Might as well have it fixed at last. Following his examination, the surgeon said, "You have bilateral hernias, something that happens about a quarter of the time, a small one on the right, which you might not have noticed, and the big one on the left." While F.G. was pulling up his pants, the surgeon, looking up from the medical record, shook his head. "You really lead an active life. I'm a little surprised. Must be uncomfortable—the hernia, I mean." F.G. smiled weakly, but said nothing. He had known about the hernia on the left; the one on the right surprised him. "If you want, we can do them both at the same operation," proposed the surgeon.

"Well . . . okay, I guess. That's what I came for."

A couple of hours after he awoke from his operation, F.G. was taken back to the operating room; the wound had filled with blood. Under local anesthesia the surgeon evacuated the blood, tied off a couple of bleeding points, then restitched the wound. This, the only immediate complication, didn't slow F.G.'s recovery. He resumed his active life, felt better about it—no longer did he double over when he coughed. Then four years after the operation, he began to notice a burning sensation in his right groin, the side that he had believed to be normal before the first operation. A lump appeared—a recurrence! This angered F.G. Why him? He had been careful, exercised to strengthen his abdominal muscles, kept his weight down.

F.G. lived in California now, a long way from his first surgeon, so after talking to a doctor acquaintance, he found a new surgeon in a nearby city who claimed to specialize in hernia repairs. This surgeon had published articles on hernia in the medical literature and reported a low recurrence rate.

After F.G.'s second operation the surgeon explained that the supposed recurrence was actually an untreated "indirect" hernia rather than a breakdown of the original repair. Apparently it had been there all the time, missed at the first operation; a congenital defect, said the surgeon, that had finally manifested itself this late in life. When last seen, two years after this second operation, F.G.'s groin was still free of hernia; he was still jogging, still trying to stay young.

The surgical community has had abundant experience with hernia: Its repair is their most frequent general surgery operation; they learn surgery by repairing hernias; they make their living doing the operation. But despite their experience, their repairs fail more often than you might expect.

If you do have a hernia and your doctor has recommended surgery, you probably need a repair—we have no good alternatives. So, go ahead, but be sure that you really have a hernia, that you are in good physical condition (cough-free and ideal weight), and that you find a technically competent surgeon.

INCIDENCE

About 15 of every 1,000 Americans, a total of over 3 million, have hernias, 518,000 of which are operated upon each year (Nyhus and Bombeck, 1986). Seventy-five percent of them occur in the lower abdomen (inguinal hernia), and another 6 percent appear just below the abdomen at the very upper end of the thigh (femoral hernia). Hernias at the site of previous abdominal operations (a late surgical complication) and umbilical (belly button) hernias account for about 13 percent of the total, and miscellaneous types make up the rest. Because they are by far the most common and important, I shall deal primarily with inguinal hernias, an affliction of men (86 percent in males). Femoral hernias, by the way, though nearby anatomically, are found mostly (84 percent) in women.

HISTORY

As early as 340 B.C. surgeons had cut into a hernia to relieve a bowel obstruction caused by the hernia, but not until the nineteenth century did they understand the structure of a hernia and the mechanism of the obstruction (Wangensteen, 1978). Early in that century, anatomists studied the complex structure of the lower abdominal wall and named the components that permit passage of the spermatic cord through the abdominal wall but hold back the abdominal organs. At that time clinicians proposed treatments less sophisticated than the anatomical concepts they were developing. For example, a Dr. Cooper, when discussing enemas in a book on hernia, said, "It is a most unpardonable neglect in the practitioner not to use tobacco [in the enema] in strangulated hernia, which ought to be impressed on the mind of every surgeon." The strangulated hernia he referred to is a hernia in which the intestine is caught in the hernia, so that its blood has become obstructed and it becomes gangrenous. When it reaches that irreversible stage, it won't respond to tobacco or to anything else except emergency surgery.

A better solution was to repair the hernia before strangulation set in. Surgeons couldn't accomplish this until anesthesia, hemostasis, and antisepsis inaugurated modern surgery. Then in 1884 Edoardo Bassini, of Padua, Italy, described the first modern, anatomically reasonable hernia repair. Many repairs have followed Bassini's and like his, were usually named after the surgeon who proposed them.

ANATOMY AND THE CAUSE OF HERNIA

A hernia of the abdominal wall is a failure of its layers to contain the abdominal viscera (the intestines and other intra-abdominal organs). Should you have a hernia, the viscera don't pour out on the floor, but they do protrude through gaps in the strong muscular and fibrous layers of the abdominal wall, until they are restrained in their migration by the skin and the fatty tissues just beneath the skin. To understand this, think of the abdominal viscera as normally contained in a sac. The anterior (front) wall of this sac consists of three main layers: The inner layer is a thin, shiny, elastic membrane called the peritoneum. The middle layer consists of muscles, which give strength and form to the abdomen; complex in structure, particularly in the lower abdomen, this muscular layer is anchored to bones and other muscles, and defects in it are what cause hernias—inguinal, umbilical, and others. The third, outer, layer of the abdominal wall is the skin and the fatty tissues just beneath it.

Both the inner (peritoneal) and the outer (skin) layers are stretchable. After a middle-layer defect develops, the viscera, which are under some pressure, press out through the defect, carrying the inner layer with them as a hernial "sac." The outer layer will stretch too, producing a bulge at the site of the hernia. The hernia itself, to repeat, is due to a defect in the middle layer.

Hernias appear in the male groin because the spermatic cord must pass through the middle layer on its way from the testicle to the outlet of the bladder. The site of passage, or "ring," is a potential defect in the abdominal wall. Femoral hernias appear nearby, but they are unrelated to the spermatic cord. They show up at the site where the major artery and vein of the leg pass into the upper thigh. At both of these sites of passage, that of the spermatic chord and that of the leg blood vessels, the enclosing abdominal wall must snug up around the passing structures, in order to restrain the abdominal contents. But the anatomical mechanisms that bring about this snugging-up are not perfect.

Furthermore, events during fetal development may set the stage for an inguinal hernia. Before birth the testicle migrates from a location within the abdomen out through the abdominal wall by the same path—the inguinal canal—that the spermatic cord will take to reach its termination in the scrotum. The testicle brings with it the spermatic cord (consisting of the vas deferens and the blood supply of the testicle), and sometimes it also carries along a narrow outpouching of the peritoneum as well. This outpouching—a congenital defect—may become the site of an indirect inguinal hernia.

Thus, since they are congenital defects, indirect hernias appear more often in the young, but not in the young exclusively (see F.G.'s case history above). And indirect hernias, by following the path of the testicle, may end up in the scrotum. Not the direct hernia. The direct hernia (the second main type of inguinal hernia) may start with a congenital weakness of the abdominal wall, but strain and aging are needed to complete it. Instead of following a course along the inguinal canal, as the indirect hernia does, the direct hernia protrudes through the back wall of the inguinal canal.

If you'd like to learn more about the anatomy of this region before having your hernia repaired, you'll find a beautifully illustrated description in a textbook entitled *Hernia* by L. M. Nyhus and R. E. Condon (1978). But even with good illustrations and a lucid text, you'll have trouble visualizing the anatomy without hands-on experience. Two-dimensional illustrations and careful prose fail to describe the three-dimensional anatomical actuality, and the feel of tissues cannot be illustrated. Trained surgeons may sometimes have a hard time identifying the detailed anatomy of this region accurately. Their failure explains some of the recurrences and some other troubles they may get into.

Robert T., a twenty-seven-year-old man, spent almost three hours in the operating room having his right inguinal hernia repaired. That evening when the chief of surgery at the hospital stopped by the postoperative recovery room, Nurse Carlson called his attention to Robert's right leg. "It's too cold," she said. It was white as a codfish and as cold as the bedpost. The chief was unable to reach the surgeon who had done the operation, but, luckily, in the doctor's lounge he found a vascular surgeon.

They examined Robert together, presently had him sent back to the operating room, where they went to work. The femoral artery (the main artery to the leg) had been tied off. A shocking technical blunder, but blunders, sometimes unrecognized at the time by their perpetrators, and rarely completely reported, *do* occur. They removed this tie and a damaged segment in order to reconnect the ends of the artery. The right leg regained its color and warmth promptly.

Before closing the wound, the vascular surgeon inspected the site of the hernia. "What do you think? I guess we might as well repair the hernia too." So they did that. Robert's postoperative recovery following this second operation was smooth.

The contents of a hernia sac usually slip back into the abdomen when you lie down or when you press on the sac with your hand. In that case, the hernia can be "reduced." But in hernias with narrow necks—indirect inguinal, femoral, or umbilical hernias usually—the contents may become stuck in the sac. The hernia is "incarcerated"—this is an emergency. Unless the hernia is reduced promptly by some means, perhaps by emergency surgery, the blood supply of the enclosed bowel will suffer, and the hernia will become "strangulated." Strangulated bowel may leak or perforate to cause peritonitis. But even before things have gone this far, the incarceration may cause intestinal obstruction, in itself a potentially lethal complication. Though less frequent today, in 1967 intestinal obstruction caused by hernia was one of the ten leading causes of death in the United States (Nyhus and Bombeck, 1986).

DIAGNOSIS

Diagnosis is made on physical exam, with one of the examiner's fingers poking uncomfortably in the groin: "Turn your head and cough." In most cases, diagnosis should require no X rays or special studies. The diagnostician may have difficulty, however, in telling an indirect from a direct inguinal hernia. This uncertainty doesn't matter if surgery is to be done, for the diagnosis can be made precisely when the area is surgically exposed. If the hernia is small or just a "weakness," diagnosticians may disagree. Is it a hernia or not? Encountering that kind of indecision, you might decline surgery. However, if it is a femoral hernia, even a small one, it is best to have surgery, because small femoral hernias have a tendency to incarcerate.

Maybe the lump down there in the private regions of your groin is something else altogether. Some examples: inflamed lymph nodes, a varicose vein, a testicle out of place, an abscess, or a cystlike structure called a hydrocele. Almost any diagnosis done cautiously can become a complex exercise. The surgeon, of course, is inclined to push ahead, settle the matter at the operating table.

INDICATIONS FOR SURGERY

If your hernia is incarcerated or strangulated, you won't be reading this book. Those hernia complications are surgical emergencies. The risk of becoming an emergency is a principal reason for having surgery on indirect inguinal, femoral, or umbilical hernias, even when they may be causing few symptoms. Direct hernias, on the other hand, have a broad-necked sac and don't incarcerate. With them discomfort is the main indication for surgery, but, as I said, the surgeon may not be able to tell whether the hernia is direct or indirect until he operates.

If your doctor is quite sure that your hernia is direct, if you have never had trouble reducing it, and if it causes you no symptoms, you can postpone surgery with little risk. The disease advances only slowly, but all untreated hernias do grow. I've seen indirect inguinal hernias (in mental-hospital patients) that grew slowly over the years until they finally reached the knees, carrying most of the intestine with them and leaving a very flat abdomen. We used to speak of the intestines in such enormous hernias as having lost their "right of abdominal domain." How could you stuff them all back into the abdominal cavity?—not enough space. The diaphragm would be pushed up, and the patient might succumb to breathing failure. Nowadays most groin hernias are submitted to repair long before they reach the knees.

If your hernia is ready for repair, be warned that obesity and chronic cough are contraindications to hernia surgery. A surgeon, when he stitches the muscles and ligaments together, finds that fat, a very weak tissue, gets in the way, resulting in a weak repair. Take the time to lose weight before having the operation. Excessive coughing increases intra-abdominal pressure in spasms, which may tear the repair apart. If you cough, perhaps you should give up smoking long before undergoing surgery. If you ignore these precautions, recurrence of the condition is likely.

Because of their tendency to incarcerate, all femoral hernias need repair. In contrast, almost no umbilical hernias in infants and young children need surgical repair. They disappear by the age of five or six, sometimes earlier, without any treatment whatsoever.

THE OPERATION

Chester McVay, a surgeon well known in the craft of hernia repair, has said, "In the entire history of surgery, no subject has been so controversial as the repair of groin hernias." The century since Bassini's first modern operation has produced so many techniques for repair that it sometimes seems as if every surgeon who has done more than a dozen of these operations has figured out his own way of going about it. Once he gets up to a hundred cases or so, he publishes, always claiming good results. Looking at this kind of data, a critic has a hard time telling if one technical variation is better than another: What kind of suture material should be used? What layers should be sewed to what? When should plastic mesh be used? and so forth.

Be that as it may, common experience, apparent success, and wide acceptance, if not absolutely convincing scientific evidence, support a few principles of hernia repair. The repair must be anatomically sound, and it must make good use of strong, normal tissues. In indirect hernia the sac must be removed. Technically the operation must be meticulous, aseptic, and finished with a bloodless field. Early ambulation following surgery has now also become an established principle.

In females, surgeons divide the round ligament, analogue of the male spermatic cord, and by doing so obtain a firm repair. Inguinal hernia recurrence among females is almost unknown. Occasionally surgeons do the same kind of repair in old men with multiple recurrences: They divide the spermatic cord in order to make a strong repair—accepting a shrunken testicle as the trade-off.

When hernia repair is done as an emergency for incarcerated or strangulated bowel, the operation may require bowel resection plus measures to relieve intestinal obstruction and treatment for peritonitis; thereby surgery becomes complex and risky.

RISKS, COMPLICATIONS

Emergency surgery for strangulated hernia has a 15 percent mortality and a 60 percent complication rate. In contrast, with elective surgery, the complication rate is 5 percent, and the mortality is described in one surgical textbook as being "negligible." Large series have been reported with no deaths.

J.B., a distinguished businessman, sat next to me at a banquet. When an equally distinguished surgeon rose to speak about the need for funds to build a new hospital wing, J.B. leaned over and whispered, "He may be your friend, but the bastard took one of my nuts, and I'll never forgive him for that. To hell with the hospital."

"What? . . . What do you mean?"

J.B. said no more then, but I talked to him a bit later. The distinguished surgeon had simply repaired J.B.'s hernia; he had not "taken" the testicle—at least not intentionally. After surgery, however, the testicle on the side of the operation had become swollen and tender, then it slowly shrank until little more than a nubbin was left. Catastrophe!

I knew how that distinguished surgeon repaired hernias. He closed the opening through which the spermatic cord passes as tightly as possible to reduce the chance of recurrence. Because he wanted to do an especially good job for his friend and possible patron, the distinguished surgeon apparently trimmed off a little more of the testicle's blood supply than usual in order to make the opening even smaller than usual. As the surgeon intended, the hernia repair was strong and enduring, but for that victory the testicle died.

The common complications following hernia repair are respiratory troubles, wound infection (1 percent), urinary retention, black-and-blue scrotum, a missed hernia (one of the causes of recurrence—see F.G.'s case), swollen testicle, and finally the shrunken testicle that became J.B.'s bitter fate.

RESULTS

Recurrence is the problem. Although millions of patients have been cured by various popular techniques, as L. M. Nyhus (1986), writing in one of the best-known surgical texts, says: "Until this subject [the matter of recurrence] is taken seriously, 100,000 patients per year will continue to be disappointed by the recurrence of what was thought to be a simple problem."

Nyhus' figure implies that 17 percent of hernia repairs fail. (When he wrote, 585,000 repairs were being done a year.) He may be right; the recurrence rate may be as high as he says, but the "reported" incidence of recurrence is published as something like this: 1 to 7 percent for indirect inguinal hernias, 4 to 10 percent for direct inguinal hernias, 1 to 7 percent for femoral hernias, and 5 to 35 percent for recurrent hernias (Nyhus and Condon, 1978). Of course the "reported" incidence is on only a small proportion of all the operations done in the United States, and the cases reported are those from busy clinics with experienced operators. Doubtless the general incidence of recurrence *is* higher than the "reported" incidence. It is surely much higher than anyone would like to have it.

Most surgeons have a high success rate with small indirect inguinal hernias. Large indirect and direct inguinal hernias cause the trouble. In the United States the best results with these have been described by Chester McVay, of Yankton, South Dakota, who reports a 3.6 percent overall recurrence rate. On the basis of McVay's record, many surgeons now use his style of repair for large indirect and direct hernias.

To outclass McVay, however, the Shouldice Hospital in Toronto, Canada, has reported even better results: a recurrence rate of only 0.6 percent after 13,108 primary inguinal hernia repairs (Glassow, 1978). Despite their impressive record, relatively few surgeons have adopted their technique. McVay considers it to be anatomically unsound and procedurally overactive. Nyhus thinks it may use too much suture material.

An important lesson from this discussion of hernia recurrence: Choose a surgeon with experience. Hernia repair may be a surgeon's first operation, the one he learns early, but unless he takes it seriously, acquires experience with it, and keeps doing it, he may never master it.

ALTERNATIVES

Some hernias, the indirect inguinal in particular, are congenital and unpreventable, but you may be able to prevent other hernias by physical conditioning and care in lifting. Avoid constipation too—it seems to bring on some hernias—and urinary straining which seems to bring on others.

Once you have a hernia, there are no good alternatives to surgery. At one time sclerosing solutions were injected around the neck of a hernial sac with the objective of getting the neck to scar down and finally close off. The neck had to be small to begin with, multiple injections were required, and strong repairs were unlikely. I haven't heard anyone advocate the technique recently.

You might get by with no special treatment. Just hold it in with your hand when you cough; don't worry if your wife grimaces. But if your hernia causes discomfort, and you want to avoid surgery, a truss may help.

A firm pad aligned over the hernial defect after the hernia has been reduced substitutes for your supporting hand, and a waist belt stiffened by a steel band holds the pad in place. Trusses tend to slip, unfortunately, or cause skin irritation where they press, and they are hard to keep clean. Furthermore, unless you can easily reduce the hernia, they don't work.

13

Backache—Slipped Disk

We have doubtless endured backache since our ancestors dropped out of the trees and started roaming the African savannah upright. If it has beset you, as it does about 80 percent of the population during an adult lifetime, you must by now have found company. Victims linked in this common plight tell each other how it goes, what to do. Listen of course, but if they recommend surgery, or if your doctor recommends surgery for your aching back, be on guard. Most victims of this ubiquitous complaint don't need surgery.

Clarence A. had played football in high school, but now at age thirty-two he no longer exercised, or at least not much. Maybe he was a little overweight, 10 pounds, say. When his wife asked him to trim the vines growing on the side of the house one Saturday afternoon, he grumbled, but he hauled out the extension ladder and went to work. After he had trimmed all he could reach and had to move the ladder, he climbed down, but with an easy carelessness that might have suited a teenager, but not him. On the lowest rung he slipped, caught his foot, and fell, twisting his back. At first he thought he might have broken his ankle, but when he tried to roll over, an excruciating flash struck him in his lower back. "Madge!"

By Monday he could still barely make it to the bathroom. Madge packed him in the car, and off they went to their clinic where, after tottering from the wheelchair to the examination table, Clarence found himself in the hands of an orthopedic surgeon he had never met before. The doctor asked him to bend, but he couldn't bend very far in any direction. The doctor's examination annoyed and hurt him, but he discovered one interesting thing during it: Coughing produced a stab of pain in his lower back which shot down the back of his right leg—strange connections among the parts of his body.

In the hospital, where he spent most of his time flat on his back on a stiff bed, he underwent a painless examination by an enormous instrument, the CAT scanner (computer assisted tomography, or computed axial tomography). This examination, the doctor had explained, would give them detailed, internal pictures of his lower back. The pictures showed that he had a slipped disk. A little of the cartilage that normally acts as a cushion between the bodies of adjacent vertebrae had been squeezed out, apparently by the fall. It pressed on spinal nerves, the doctor said, causing pain. But with rest, things would quiet down, then with physiotherapy and a graded exercise schedule that would strengthen his back, they would return him almost to normal. He'd have to be more careful in the future.

Clarence spent two weeks in the hospital, five weeks at home resting most of the time but returning to the hospital for physiotherapy, where he had hot baths, gentle massage, and assisted walking. Two months after the injury he was back at the job, but he couldn't sit still for long. At home he felt better pacing the floor then he did slouching in front of the TV. How about surgery for the slipped disk? Not necessary, at least not now, said the surgeon. In the future, who could tell?

During the last fifty years surgeons have won a share of the profitable backache trade with an operation, the slipped disk operation—done now at the rate of 230,000 a year in this country—that helps many patients. If your backache is caused by a slipped disk, you may need the operation. But backache has a diverse set of often poorly understood causes, and there are ways other than surgery with which to treat the slipped disk. Recovery may require no active treatment, only time.

Low back pain is usually a self-limiting complaint, but it costs at least $16 billion a year and disables 5.4 million Americans (Frymoyer 1988; "Diagnostic and therapeutic," 1989). Perhaps 80 percent of the population will suffer at least one episode during an active adult life; thus, it has become the most common cause of long-term disability in persons, under age forty-five. The average age of patients undergoing surgery for a slipped disk is forty-two. Rare before age fifteen and uncommon after sixty, it disables active workers who seek both compensation and cure. In most sufferers the affliction is poorly understood and doubtless complicated but benign. Only about 1 percent of patients with acute backache have the signs of a slipped disk. Backache acquires economic impact and public attention because of psychological, legal, and social features.

Prior to 1934 millions of victims must have recovered without surgery. Then at that time, the slipped disk was identified as a cause of backache, and two surgeons devised a way of reaching the disk surgically from the back (operation called laminectomy) to remove the source of trouble. New hope for aching back victims. I remember first hearing of disk surgery in the late 1930s when a visiting surgeon from the Mayo Clinic lectured about his remarkable experience. He showed us special X rays of the spinal canal after dye had been injected that demonstrated disks protruding where they shouldn't be, and photographs of the specimens he had removed. Before this lecture I had been taught that "sciatica" was likely an "inflammation" of the sciatic nerve. Here instead was something rational and demonstrable.

During the ensuing years surgeons have modified the operation to make it less traumatic, and they have refined their indications for surgery, but their basic objective remains the same: Locate the bits of cartilagelike material that have been squeezed out from between two adjacent vertebrae and remove them.

At forty-three Bert D. was suffering his second attack of disabling low backache. The first attack had laid him low for several weeks about six years previously. The doctor had said then that he thought it was a torn ligament, but he couldn't be absolutely sure. There had been a tender spot, deep in the muscles, lower than the kidney, Bert thought, on the left side.

This time the pain had started when he was lifting a box of books. It was on the left side again, but now different and worse. When he moved— tried to walk for example—a stab of pain shot down the back of his leg all the way to the knee, sometimes lower. He had a CAT scan; the first time, plain X rays had shown nothing, but now, said the neurosurgeon to whom

Bert had been referred, the CAT scan showed a definite ruptured disk on the left.

Almost two weeks in the hospital, and the pain was no better as far as Bert could tell, so he agreed readily when the neurosurgeon recommended surgery—a pretty clear-cut case. They would do a microdiskectomy under general anesthesia—only a small incision from which Bert would recover promptly. Immediately after the surgery his back hurt more than ever, but he noticed that the pain that had shot down the back of his leg, the pain they had called sciatica, was gone. A month after surgery Bert was back at the office, and by three months he was just about cured.

NATURE OF THE DISEASE

Many injuries or anomalies cause low back pain: bruise, torn ligament, strain, fracture, arthritis, cancer, congenital defect, infection, spondylolisthesis (one vertebra slides ahead of the others because of a deficiency in its moorings), osteoporosis, and degenerative disease (deterioration of disks due to aging), to list a few. Pain may be "referred" to the back from disease in other parts of the body, such as the large intestine, the heart, or the kidney. In an individual patient, the cause may remain obscure, and since a complaint of pain is subjective, the examiner may have difficulty pinpointing the source of trouble and assessing its intensity.

The examiner's problems are accentuated by the patient's problems—emotional, psychological, and money. Persons with low back pain often view their occupations as boring, repetitive, and dissatisfying, and this causes depression, anxiety, hypochondriasis, alcoholism, marriage breakup, headache, and ulcer. Patients involved with legal claims or workmen's compensation for their aching back tend to have a slow recovery; because of this, in published reports of treatment, their results may be considered separately.

But when the trouble *is* a slipped disk (variously called lumbar disk herniation, prolapsed lumbar disk, disk protrusion, disk disease, or lumbar intervertebral disk prolapse), it means that a strain, such as heavy lifting, has squeezed some of the cartilagelike disk (the nucleus pulposus) out from between two adjacent vertebrae into the spinal canal where it may then press on spinal nerves to cause pain and perhaps other disabilities such as muscle weakness. A nerve root irritated at one point becomes irritable along its length. The usual location of the prolapse is at the fourth or fifth lumbar vertebra (lower back, just above the pelvis). Once ruptured, a disk never regains normal position, but the protrusion may miss the nerves, and, in any case, the deformity usually becomes quite well tolerated after a while.

In a typical clinical history, the first acute attack of lower back pain, occurring between ages thirty and fifty, is followed in later attacks by radiating pain—sciatica—that shoots down the back of the thigh. Occupations that require heavy lifting in the forward-bent position or exposure to vibrations are usually thought to increase risk, but in some series of cases, no particular style of work has stood out as predisposing. Slipped disk is prevalent in males over females at a ratio of 1.4 to 1.

DIAGNOSIS

If the pain settles in the lower back, not radiating down the leg, there could, as noted above, be various causes; but radiating pain that follows the course of lumbar nerves or the course of the sciatic nerve down the leg (the reason it's called sciatica) characterizes a slipped disk. Changes in nerve function, other than pain, show up as altered reflexes, muscle weakness, spinal curvature, and poor urine or bowel control. These signs and symptoms all point to the diagnosis of a slipped disk, but the diagnosis should be confirmed by special x-ray examination.

A high-resolution CAT scan (computer assisted tomography) provides the diagnostic key. Prior to the CAT scanner, in a technique called myelography, special dyes were injected into the spinal canal or into the disk itself before X ray. Since it delineates the slipped disk directly without the dye, the modern CAT scan has replaced myelography, except for borderline cases.

Remember, no diagnostic technique can incontrovertibly link the symptoms with the findings to make an absolute diagnosis. Diagnosis is almost always an exercise in probability.

Other causes of backache such as arthritis, tumor, or spondylolithesis (forward displacement of one vertebra over another) may explain the pain, or with one of these a slipped disk may appear to furnish a compound cause. In most cases the cause is never accurately specified; among persons with acute low back pain, only 10 to 20 percent can be given a precise anatomical diagnosis. Facing this uncertainty, doctors may still feel obliged to state a diagnosis, whether or not they are sure of what is wrong. If you want to know where you stand, or if surgery is recommended, ask for the evidence.

INDICATIONS FOR SURGERY

Without a precise pathological-anatomical diagnosis, surgery isn't indicated, and probably no more than 5 to 10 percent of patients with unrelenting sciatica—radiating pain in a nerve distribution—eventually require surgery (Frymoyer, 1988). Surgery is neither necessary nor effective for the rest. If pain is intolerable and unrelieved, or if neurological defects are severe—foot drop, as an example—surgery may be indicated early. Otherwise, accept conservative treatment for perhaps as long as three months. If it fails, and a slipped disk is evident on CAT scan, surgery may then be your best choice. But there are other alternatives—see below.

THE OPERATION

Some years ago surgeons might have used muscle strippings, tenotomies (dividing tendons), fasciotomies (cutting through sheets of fibrous tissue), and fusions of the sacroiliac joints, but these operations have lost out. This branch of surgery, too, has its list of abandoned operations.

Later, surgeons would consider one of three operative possibilities for backache: a fusion of the lumbar vertebrae with bone grafts, excision of the protruded disk, or a combination of fusion and disk excision. In the long competitive struggle between orthopedic surgeons and neurosurgeons for these cases, the orthopedic surgeons captured the fusions, and they shared the disk excisions with the neurosurgeons, perhaps seizing most of them.

In time fusion was abandoned. Disk excision survived, first, as an operation called a laminectomy (removal of a part of the bony arch of the spinal canal to get at the disk) and then, more recently, as a less traumatic operation with a smaller incision. In something called a microdiskectomy (Bert D.'s operation) the operator uses an incision only about an inch long and magnification with an operating microscope in order to get at the disk without removing any bone. Its advocates claim that it is as effective as the bigger operation. It may well be.

Now available is an operation called manual percutaneous diskectomy, done blindly through a tube, and an even more elegant technique called automatic percutaneous lumbar diskectomy ("Diagnostic and therapeutic," 1989). This one, also a blind operation, is done with a long blunt needle, having at its end a clever pumping, cutting, and sucking mechanism. The manufacturer of the (disposable) instrument says that surgeons are doing this operation at the rate of 1,000 a month. What next? Lasers, of course. Tests in dogs have been reported. Surgery has a tendency to become technically more stylish, neater, safer, and sometimes even more effective, but, as is usually the case, none of these newer techniques has passed the test of a random, controlled clinical study. In fact, published reports, even without control, are rare.

RESULTS

Surgical mortality is low. One expert reported over 7,000 disk cases with only one fatality (Simmons, 1980). Infection, as you might expect, is always a risk, and in this kind of surgery the operator may inadvertently injure nerves. Hemorrhage may complicate recovery, and a chronic postoperative inflammation (arachnoiditis) may explain some of the poor late results. Postoperative disability lasts from six weeks to three months— longer, by the way, than the disability associated with successful conservative therapy.

Satisfactory relief has been realized in about 85 percent of patients. Pain shooting down the leg (sciatica) responds well to surgery; pain in the back responds less predictably. There are late failures. If the pain continues or recurs, it may be attributed to rupture of an adjacent disk, extrusion of additional fragments, failure to find the ruptured disk, damage to a nerve root, adhesions, or inflammation. Or maybe the patient has the same vague, undiagnosed cause he first appeared with.

In compensation cases results are poor. An article by English surgeons (Shannon and Paul, 1979) points out that "There are numerous reputable authors who suggest compensation claims as one reason for long-term failure of disk operations." Someone who is getting money for his injured back is consciously or unconsciously reluctant to give up the cash by an admission that his back is now perfectly okay. Therefore, surgeons try to avoid operating on compensation cases. Other evidence supports the importance of psychology in the outcome. Saline injections, for instance, as a control for the chymopapain injections I will discuss later, worked in 40 percent of cases. Here, as with any surgery used primarily to treat pain, the placebo effect of surgery decidedly improves the results.

Without a sham operation as control for a clinical test, the placebo effect cannot be usefully estimated. No one has tested disk surgery against a sham operation, but Henrik Weber of Oslo, Norway, reported a randomized clinical comparison of conservative and surgical treatment for patients with uncertain indications for surgery in 1983 (Weber). The 280 patients, all of whom had clinical and x-ray evidence of a slipped disk, were divided into three groups: those who beyond a doubt required surgical therapy, those with no indications for surgery who were then treated conservatively, and finally a group of 126 patients with uncertain indications. After fourteen days in the hospital, the patients in this last group still had some pain and a few physical findings. Among them surgical or conservative therapy was chosen by randomization. The surgically treated patients had a statistically significant better result at the one-year-follow-up examination, but the difference was no longer statistically significant after four years. "Back insufficiency" was their main complaint at the final examination, equally distributed in the two treatment groups.

Weber noted that in the nonoperated group, 25 percent of the patients were cured and 36 percent showed satisfactory improvement. If these patients, approximately 60 percent of the total, had been submitted to surgery, they would have had an unnecessary surgical procedure, he said, but he did not describe how to recognize them before surgery.

CHEMONUCLEOLYSIS, THE CHEMICAL ALTERNATIVE

Sarah L. couldn't return to work. When her backache had started, her doctor had said to rest. Okay, with that she could comply; she didn't feel like doing anything else. But now three weeks had gone by, and she felt no better. On the doctor's recommendation she had gone to a physiotherapist whose heat treatments and massage felt good, but her back still ached. Sometimes the pain radiated down through her right buttock to the back of her thigh.

Now she was in the hospital where they had done a CAT scan that confirmed the diagnosis of slipped disk. Sarah hated to think of surgery, but she was coming around to acceptance, until the orthopedic surgeon said that he thought they could use a new treatment—injection of a solution directly into the slipped disk in order to shrink it. She didn't like needles, but the surgeon said the injection would be done under general anesthesia. Before we go ahead, he said, it was important that she not be pregnant. Okay on that score—Sarah was forty-eight. Any sensitivity to drugs or medicines? No, she'd never had allergies.

Sarah had the injection of an enzyme called chymopapain. By the time she left the hospital, four days after the injection, her back still ached— worse, she believed, than it had before the injection—and her back was stiff—muscle spasm, they said. The spasm lasted for a couple of weeks, but then gradually worked its way out. By six weeks she was back at work, no longer thinking much about her back.

Injection of an enzyme extracted from the latex of the papaya tree (chymopapain) into the disk has become an alternative to surgery. It acts on the cartilage of the nucleus pulposus (the center of the disk), destroying its water-binding capacity. As the disk loses water, it shrinks, thereby, presumably, drawing in the extruded protrusions which were pressing on the nerves and causing pain and disability.

A candidate for injection should have a clear-cut disk protrusion and pain that has persisted, despite at least four weeks of conservative treatment. Under local or general anesthesia a long needle (two long needles if there are two slipped disks) is inserted into the disk under careful fluoroscopic, x-ray control. Dye is injected first, more X rays, and then if everything is okay, the chymopapain is injected. In clinical use, without controlled testing, 70 percent of patients have had good results.

But chymopapain is a drug, and unlike surgery it comes under the control of the FDA, which, in their usual fashion, insisted on random, controlled clinical tests before approval (Sampson, 1978; Gunby, 1983). Very well, let's have the tests. To the dismay of chymopapain's enthusiastic supporters, the controlled tests showed that the placebo worked as well as the drug. No approval.

Something must be wrong! A few supporters said that the placebo solution, which was not just saltwater (it had some of the chemicals found in the chymopapain solution, but not the chymopapain), was itself an effective treatment. They even gave the placebo a name, CEI. (Wags called it "placeboase.") But the drug company took the matter seriously and patented CEI. Years went by, the drug company seemed to lose interest in seeking FDA approval, but crusaders led by Dr. Lyman Smith of Chicago, who had devised the technique and watched it become popular in Canada and other places, kept trying. "How come," he asked, "the drug is safe and effective in Toronto—and not here?"

Finally a second randomized, double-blind control test was started, and this one came out okay, in favor of chymopapain (Javid et al., 1983). Patients followed for six months (What? Just six months?) had more failures among the placebo group (thirty-one out of fifty-three) than among the chymopapain group (fifteen out of fifty-five). With this (rather indecisive) evidence in hand, the FDA approved chymopapain in 1982. Anaphylactic shock (a severe, sometimes fatal, allergic reaction), which has caused two deaths, has been the most significant risk of the treatment.

In an unprecedented burst of cooperation between traditionally competitive organizations, the American Academy of Orthopaedic Surgeons and the American Association of Neurological Surgeons began a massive professional education program with forty courses, held in Chicago or Los Angeles, to train surgeons in the "intradiscal therapy" technique in just one day. Orthopedic surgeons, who had been losing out to neurosurgeons in the microdiskectomy business, were now quickly back into the fray (along with the neurosurgeons, of course) at about $1,000 a shot for the chymopapain treatment.

Not all are contented with this new therapy, however. Some neurosurgeons have claimed that it is less "cost-effective" than microdiskectomy, and in a prospective study with random assignment, Swedish investigators found that surgical removal of the disk was more effective than chymopapain injection (Ejeskar, 1983). In recent years, enthusiasm for chymopapain has waned because of its neurological complications, allergic reactions, and persisting muscle spasms (in 20 percent of clients) (Frymoyer, 1988).

OTHER ALTERNATIVES

If your doctor has recommended surgery for your bad back, cure is on your mind right now, not prevention, but once you are past this episode, you might, for the future, want to consider prevention: exercise, weight loss, care in lifting. A strong back resists injury. A pot belly pulls the spine out of line and into a vulnerable sag. You might not have to lift those heavy weights at all, but if you do, strength and technique count; start your lift with a squat, not a bend.

Traditional conservative treatment for acute backache, an alternative I have referred to repeatedly, consists of bed rest to begin with, pain killers, hot or cold packs, traction, then graded exercises, physical therapy, perhaps a brace support. Its most important ingredient may be time. As with any injury, this injury tends to heal, or you tend to accommodate to it—in time.

But is *rest* really the right way to develop a strong, healthy back? New evidence from Denmark advocates vigorous exercise, under supervision, for chronic low back pain (Manniche, 1988). Skip the rest, get started on the exercise right away. Tests were carried out on 105 patients, none of whom had characteristic signs of a ruptured disk, spondylolysis, or osteomalacia (softening of the bones)—they had, that is, the common kind of chronic backache. With patients randomized into three groups, the results consistently favored intensive, dynamic back exercises carried out for three months. Sounds good to me; I've been pumping a little iron for years with never a backache.

Unless your doctor has clearly demonstrated that you have a slipped disk, conservative therapy, whether rest or exercise, should be your first choice. It may be your only sensible choice. "The great secret of doctors," said Dr. Lewis Thomas, "known only to their wives, but still hidden from the public, is that most things get better by themselves; most things, in fact, are better in the morning."

It's common to think of chiropractic when you think of back. Chiropractors work on the back. I haven't had enough experience with their work to know when it might be useful for backache, but I have been told by those with more experience that in some environments chiropractic may provide the most easily available source of physiotherapy and massage—treatments that speed recovery or at least provide comfort while natural recovery takes place. Orthodox physicians will often advocate physiotherapy and massage, but they seldom carry it out themselves, nor may they be able to provide it outside of an expensive and sometimes inconvenient hospital physiotherapy department.

Chiropractic is burdened with an irrational theory that attributes disease to a "subluxation" of the spine (a partial dislocation that chiropractic advocates have never satisfactorily demonstrated), which causes pressure on the spinal nerves. In order to cure disease, they manipulate the spine to correct this (evidently nonexistent) partial dislocation. With a slipped disk you might think that they would be in hog heaven, because here finally, is a disease in which symptoms are actually caused by pressure on the spinal nerves. But a slipped disk is neither a dislocation nor a "subluxation," and, as we have seen by studying some of the mistakes that surgeons have made in other regions of the body (see section on abandoned operations, Chapter 2), bad practice follows bad theory.

Also irrational, if judged by their anatomical and physiological theory alone, are alternatives such as acupuncture and transcutaneous electric nerve stimulation. As with the more traditional treatments, however, these alternatives make use of time, our natural tendency to heal, and the placebo effect. With a subjective, self-limiting ailment such as the

common backache, ointments, incantations, frequent hugging, sympa-
thy, a vegetarian diet, sleeping with a small pillow under the back,
Tylenol, a stiff drink, a Jacuzzi (with a stiff drink), almost anything that at
the time appeals, will work. But please take it easy on the surgery.

14

Total Hip Replacement (THR)

Surgeons and engineers have joined talents to create a remarkable, effective hip replacement, better than many of us expected. THR substitutes a smoothly operating metal and plastic device for a painful joint that has been destroyed by arthritis or injury. Although difficult and occasionally beset with serious complications, the operation attains excellent early results. Later, because living tissues reject foreign bodies, in the way your finger rejects a sliver, the artificial hip loosens, and the joint becomes unstable.

If THR has been recommended to you, the operation may be a blessing; on the other hand, since the artificial joints are imperfect, you might want to postpone surgery, especially if you are young. At any age, wait until you are disabled and in pain. Engineers continue to improve these artificial joints and will have better devices in a year or two, just as the joints they have now are better than those of a couple of years ago. In this chapter I'll tell you about the operation and the limitations of an artificial joint. If you decide to have surgery, find a surgeon competent with this specific operation.

Some 2 million artificial devices are used each year to replace body parts ruined by injury or disease: a million or so eye lenses and lesser numbers of pacemakers, heart valves, and joints—more than 120,000 hip joints. Perhaps, say some medical futurists, from 1 percent to 3 percent of people reaching age sixty-five will eventually need a THR (Kelsey, 1983). Presently, 60 percent are used in persons over sixty-five, and 25 percent in the fifty-five to sixty-four decade (Consensus Conferences. Total Hip-Joint, 1982). Plainly, as with most artificial substitutions, it is an old person's operation and an indication of future need. Will future survivors have as many new parts as Alice's Tin Woodman or the Bionic Man-/Woman? Currently successful replacements, such as the artificial hip joint, are relatively simple in concept. Complex organs, such as an artificial heart, are still beyond our technical competence.

Dr. N.E., a busy surgeon, practiced standing. In his office he went from one patient to the next, on his feet all the time, and he stood for long hours in the operating room. The life suited him, but at age sixty, arthritis struck, first one hip, then the other. Soon he could hardly get around; if he walked or if he just stood, the pain frightened him. He took aspirin, bought an electric wheelchair, used two canes when he stood, but this was no way to practice surgery. He retired at age sixty-four.

In 1974, the year he retired, during a medical meeting in San Francisco, N.E. had a chance to talk to John Charnley of England, the originator of the modern THR operation. Time to have the operation, said Charnley, was when it got so bad you couldn't go any more. "Those who have advanced disease get better results, generally, than those with less advanced disease. Wait. But when you are ready, if you want to come to England, I'll do it." He warned N.E. against using alcohol and narcotics in the meantime. Physicians with arthritis seem especially prone to addiction, he said. He took N.E. by the shoulders, looked him in the eye: "Don't you do that!"

Dr. N.E. avoided addiction, tried to control his pain with analgesics and rest. But a couple of years after he saw Charnley, he knew he was ready for surgery, and he went to a large American clinic. There they said he was overweight. He had to lose 25 pounds before they did his first THR in 1977. When he awoke after the operation, the pain in that hip was gone. Immediate relief! Same thing after the opposite hip was replaced three months later. Pain gone, no complications. Though N.E. had had some coronary heart disease and high blood pressure, he recovered promptly from both operations.

Ten years after the operations he says: "I'm not brand new. I don't walk at great lengths, and I have these other problems, which I know are results of aging and not complications of the operations. I get angina, I've become a mild sort of diabetic, and I have some peripheral vascular disease. My legs aren't all that great. . . . But as for getting about and into my car and going someplace, I can do that. I don't go for hikes obviously. You can live a long time and never play golf." Of the surgeons who replaced his hips he says, "I'll love 'em forever."

After decades of inadequate stainless steel ball-and-socket installations, pins, and plates for the hip, the modern THR appeared in the late 1950s, a result of the engineering and operative innovations of John Charnley of Lancashire, England, the surgeon whom Dr. N.E. had seen in San Francisco. Charnley, a civil engineer as well as a surgeon, employed new materials, effective lubrication, efficient design, a cold-curing acrylic cement, and an exceptionally clean operating-room environment. Orthopedic surgeons rapidly accepted his concepts, and less rapidly learned how to perform this operation.

INDICATIONS FOR SURGERY

As an emergency operation, THR is used for hip fracture when healing seems unlikely because of the nature of the fracture and the patient's general state of health. As an elective operation, it is used for arthritis, necrosis, and failed prostheses (the operation itself creates a future need for the operation). The most common indications for THR are osteoarthritis (the arthritis of older people), 60 percent, fracture-dislocations, 11 percent, rheumatoid arthritis (the arthritis of younger people), 7 percent, aseptic (noninfectious) bone necrosis, 7 percent, and revision of previous hip operations, 6 percent (Consensus Conferences, "Total hip," 1982). Except perhaps for a fracture-dislocation, the diagnosis alone is not sufficient reason for recommending surgery. The disease must cause sufficient pain and disability in suitable candidates to justify a major operation that requires a long recovery period. As we have seen, with this as with all elective surgery, the decision must finally be yours. Do you have enough pain and disability to risk the operation and endure the comeback?

   C. B. Sledge of Boston, in advising doctors whether or not they should make a recommendation of surgery, suggests that "the near-certain success following total hip replacement [must be] considered in light of eventual possible failure in certain combinations of disease state, age, weight, and activity levels". He is saying, I think: The operation relieves pain and restores function early, but tends to fail later on.

Youth and obesity are relative contraindications. Dr. N.E. had to lose weight before his surgeons would operate. The artificial joint he would acquire is simply not strong and durable enough to carry great weight, last for a long life, or withstand the buffeting an active young person or an athlete will give it. Normal bones and joints constantly reheal and rebuild themselves as part of the living process. In striking contrast to the fixed, lifeless framework we see in a preserved skeleton, living bone changes continuously to retain or modify its form, else a child would never grow or a fracture heal. An artificial joint has *no* intrinsic rebuilding or repairing mechanism. It simply wears out, as do running shoes or faucet washers.

If the recipient may not be able to make use of his expensive new joint because of nervous system disorders, such as stroke, this, too, becomes a relative contraindication to the surgery.

THE OPERATION

The surgeon replaces both the head and the socket of the diseased hip joint with a metal and plastic substitute that will be held in place by its weight-bearing design, by the in-growth of surrounding tissues, and by glue. Muscles normally attached to the joint are wired to the prosthesis. Though the hip is not near vital organs, the preservation of which always challenges the abdominal or chest surgeon, it is deep, difficult to get at, and the focus of strong muscular forces which must be dealt with.

THR is prone to infection. Living tissues, exposed by opening a skin incision, can withstand some contamination because they are able to destroy the bacterial invaders; they do so regularly after routine surgery. Some bacteria fall into any operative wound from the operating-room air, but the white blood cells circulating through living tissue destroy them. Foreign bodies have no circulating, defensive, white-blood-cell army. If contaminated beforehand or during surgery by the operating-room environment, a prosthesis like an artificial hip may provide a retreat for bacteria, giving them time to proliferate in numbers adequate to invade the surrounding tissues successfully.

Surgeons must, at all costs, avert this disastrous scenario. They cannot convert the prosthesis into a living, self-protecting organism, so they do the next best thing—reduce the likelihood of infection by employing special clean-air operating rooms, rigorous aseptic technique, and prophylactic antibiotics.

Artificial joints tend to wear out. In their search for durable artificial joints, ingenious biomedical engineers and material scientists have used polymers such as polymethyl methacrylate and polyethylene, or carbon, or ceramics (Consensus Conferences, "Total hip," 1982). Recent models have employed wrought, isostatically hot-pressed cobalt-base alloys, chemical modifications of stainless steel, and titanium-base alloys. These complex modern materials are more compatible with human tissues than materials used in the past. There is less wear, and therefore less debris is deposited in the surrounding tissues.

How best to fix this complex device in position? Techniques for cementing it in place complete with a technique that depends on bone growth into a porous surface to hold it in place. The older models were held by cement, but concern over how many became loose started investigators on an exploration of biologically more compatible, noncemented techniques. The issue is unsettled. Said C. B. Sledge, an orthopedic surgeon and investigator, "As of today, a cemented hip is predictably excellent over a long period of time with a low failure rate. It is still the gold standard. However, the biological approach [noncement method] has to be the final solution" (Kirn, 1987c). "Final" solution? It seems unjustified to expect stability in a rapidly changing arena. Moreover, one might claim that the true "final" solution would be prevention or cure of arthritis.

RISKS, COMPLICATIONS, RESULTS

Describing the Mayo Clinic experience, D. L. Conn (1983) says, "If good medical and surgical judgment are brought to bear on the patient's behalf, the total hip arthroplasty is a remarkably safe operation, even in the aged and infirm." The mortality is 1 percent to 3 percent.

Complications: Operative complications described are fracture of the femur, nerve injury, blood vessel injury, and hemorrhage. Early postoperative complications are infection, hemorrhage, dislocation or partial dislocation of the joint, fracture, and limb-length discrepancy (that is, one leg will end up longer than the other). In addition, any patient may suffer the usual postoperative complications of any major surgery: urinary tract infection, venous inflammation and clotting (which may cause pulmonary embolism), heart attack, stroke, pneumonia, and miscellaneous respiratory troubles.

Late failures are reported in 10 percent or more of patients. One fifteen-year follow-up study, for example, concluded that all but 13 percent were still "good" or "excellent." Another found that 24 percent were "unsatisfactory" at eight years (Kirn, 1987c). Failure may show up in various ways, loosening of the implant being the most common. In some follow-up studies, mechanical loosening can be seen on X ray in 30 percent of cases, although it doesn't inconvenience every patient. By seven to ten years, loosening and need for revision is common in younger patients, in those who walk fast, and in those who are overweight. Limb-length discrepancy due to loosening may cause enough instability to require a subsequent operation.

Fracture of the prosthetic stem, caused by metal fatigue in active patients, is less common, but it requires surgery. In one study the average interval from insertion to failure because of fracture of the stem was three years, for loosening of the stem, three years, and for loosening of the head, four and a half years (Consensus Conferences, "Total hip," 1982). Of 400 failed hip and knee replacements, reported in another study, 80 percent were due to mechanical reasons and 20 percent were due to infections.

Infection, a disaster, appears in about 1 percent of patients. At the very least, the entire prosthesis must be removed, and it may not be possible ever to replace it safely, in which case the patient has a useless extremity. Infection may appear early (in 40 percent of infected cases), two to twenty-four months after surgery (45 percent), or late, two to five years after surgery (15 percent). When it appears late, it may appear in previously asymptomatic patients, or in patients with some other infection, such as a urinary-tract infection, which has been carried to the joint.

Bone buildup around the joint (another late complication), loosening of the prosthesis, and other so-called reactive complications are the consequence of the body's natural response to foreign materials. Normal tissues tend to reject large pieces of metal or plastic. The glue, too, causes reaction, as do the fine particles that wear off in use. The body must deal with these particles in some way. Elevated levels of cobalt and chromium are found in the blood and organs. P. G. Bullough (1983), of the Hospital for Special Surgery in New York, says that, "Reactions to implants should be considered the rule and not the exception. All foreign bodies are capable of producing an inflammatory reaction." He says, further, with respect to fibrosis, which is prominent in rejection and loosening of the artificial hip, that it "should be considered the universal endpoint in the body's defense mechanism against foreign material; where there is an implant, expect fibrosis."

Fibrosis, loosening, infection, or fracture may cause an artificial hip to fail; nonetheless, patients with few medical problems before surgery do surprisingly well with their artificial joints; they recover 80 percent of their normal gait over the first two to four years and have excellent relief of pain (Perrin, 1985). The new, smooth, shiny, metal substitute moves more comfortably than the crumbly, spindly, worn-out, arthritic original. Good to excellent results are reported in 90 percent of patients. Students of social efficiency say that this surgery can be cost-effective for our society if quality of life is considered. It can't be justified on purely economic grounds, however, because many of the recipients are no longer wage-earners.

Kenneth F., a retired police lieutenant and recreational tennis player, was taking an anti-inflammatory pill for a hip that pained him when he played, but the pill aggravated his peptic ulcer, which bled a little. His doctor sent him to an orthopedic surgeon who, after examining X rays, declared that Ken should have a hip transplant. "Wait a minute!" said Ken.

"Okay," said the orthopedic surgeon, "you keep playing tennis then, and when the pain gets too severe, call me, and we'll see what we can do."

The surgeon wrote Ken, stating that Ken's problem was "degenerative" arthritis. "Your condition will only be getting worse." Ken thought this over. He was sixty-eight, but he wanted to keep on playing tennis, and by now he was no longer moving well on the tennis court. He returned to the orthopedic surgeon, who, quite promptly, did a THR on Ken's right hip.

Ken wasn't able to walk much for the first two months after surgery, but by the third month he was back at the court, holding a racket, standing around. Then he started playing a little doubles. Now, four and a half years after the operation, he says, "I've been playing tennis about five days a week. After the third set, it hurts a little, but I get around a lot better than I was able to before, and the pain is much less than I've had for ten years or so. I'm very pleased with what has happened to me. . . . Of course, I can't walk very well. I can't walk rapidly. It's painful. On the court when I recover a ball after the point, I walk slowly, but I run like crazy when I play. Do you think it's psychological?"

How about loosening of the hip with all that activity? Maybe a little, the surgeon told him at the last follow-up exam, maybe some of the cement has turned to sand, but not much. It doesn't seem to worry Ken.

After two to three weeks of hospitalization and several more weeks with walking aids and physical therapy, the usual patient achieves independence in about three months. He or she is told to include all activities involved in daily living: unlimited walking, driving, dancing, and sex. Avoid repetitive activities that overload the hip such as jogging, jumping, and racket sports—all this advice individualized of course. Ken F., as we have seen, tolerates tennis quite well. Avoid excessive hip flexion as when squatting. Keep in good physical shape, eat a prudent diet, and so forth.

REVISION SURGERY

Maybe your doctor has recommended a *second* operation. Because of late failures many patients now face the prospect of revision surgery. Results don't match those of the first operation. The infection rate is twice as high, and other complications increase. Only about 60 percent have satisfactory functional results after a revision for mechanical failure (Consensus Conferences, "Total hip," 1982).

Clara P. had enough pain in her right hip to cause a slight limp. "You've got arthritis," said her internist, "nothing I can do will cure it, but these new artificial hip joints are excellent." He insisted that she see an orthopedic surgeon. "But surgery?" said Clara, "I don't think I want an operation."

Her husband, Jim, encouraged her to consider surgery, as did another doctor who was a family friend. So Clara saw an orthopedic surgeon, who took X rays, confirmed the diagnosis, and attributed her pain to the arthritis, but he didn't think she should have a hip replacement at that time. Her internist was furious. "You've got to take care of this."

He sent her to a second orthopedic surgeon who went along with the tide of opinion and replaced her hip a little over ten years ago, shortly after she had retired from her law practice. When she first tried to walk, it felt as if she "had an elephant leg attached." She fainted. But on the second try she got along with a walker, and was able to leave the hospital ten days after surgery. At home she took care of herself and helped her husband, who was then recovering from a mild stroke.

Three months following surgery the leg pained more than it had preoperatively. No problem, said the surgeon, healing takes time. The pain got worse, however. She went back again, and X rays showed that the cement had failed; the spike of the prosthesis was out of line and jamming the bone each time she took a step. Luckily the femur had not shattered.

Six months after the first operation, they inserted a second artificial hip with a new and longer spike. Unfortunately this longer spike was not inserted quite deeply enough, and the right leg became longer than the left. She limped a little. Furthermore, she had to pay for this surgery herself.

Four years ago, approximately six years after the first operation, she suffered a dislocation of the artificial joint and was hospitalized, flat in bed, for a week. Then two years ago on a Mediterranean cruise, she stepped too high when disembarking from a ship-to-shore boat and dislocated the hip again. Doctors in Venice, Italy, reduced it and encased her in a total body cast. She was shipped home "like I was in a coffin." Clara and the cast occupied three airline seats.

How is it now ten years after the first operation? She can walk two or three blocks slowly, but. . . "Of course I have very little use of joint rotation, and I have to be very careful that it doesn't go out of the socket." She is utterly cautious now, she says. She doesn't cross her legs or bring her leg up or bend over to the floor. "It's something you live with." Finally, she says, "I wouldn't recommend having this kind of surgery unless you were just totally helpless."

When revision is for infection, the outlook is worse. Not only are there mechanical difficulties; the infection must be completely controlled. Diagnosis may be difficult. If the infection involves the prosthesis, the prosthesis must be removed. If implantation of another THR is to be considered, usually this must be delayed, for months or years, until complete healing.

ALTERNATIVES

No randomized, controlled clinical study to compare THR with other treatments has been undertaken, nor are any contemplated—an obvious shortcoming, but one hard to rectify as long as the operation remains in continuous flux. A five-year test completed now would have told us only about a now obsolete operation. THR is still, in a sense, an experimental operation: Surgeons and engineers have settled on neither the best prosthesis nor the best way to use the prosthesis. Because poor late results keep coming in, they are not likely to do so soon. This surgery is another example of a "halfway technology": a complex treatment that is the best we can provide until effective prevention or a curative treatment becomes possible.

No specific agents are available to prevent, retard, or reverse osteoarthritis. Drugs—aspirin for example—may reduce pain and minimize the consequences of inflammation, but they don't halt the disease. Systemic steroid therapy—once thought to be the great hope—has side effects that outweigh its benefits. Steroids injected in the joint may help, however.

Many patients with osteoarthritis can be managed for a long time without drugs. Proper rest and protective devices, such as canes, crutches, and walkers, come into use. Included, too, are weight reduction and physical therapy programs designed to relieve pain, restore joint motion, and develop muscular strength. Sex counseling and vocational advice fit into a comprehensive program.

Surgical alternatives to THR are simpler, but still major, operations that restore less function than does a successful THR. You end up with a limp and maybe only walker or wheelchair mobility. Technically these operations are usually divisions and realignments (osteotomies) of the femur and pelvis, designed to direct weight bearing away from the diseased joint. Rarely used now as primary operations, they may be used after a failed THR when something is desperately needed, and when no sensible surgeon wants to try putting in another artificial joint.

15

The Eye

"O loss of sight," wrote John Milton the poet, "of thee I most complain!" He might have had his sight restored (and the character of his poetry changed) had he lived in this century rather than the seventeenth. Eye surgery has transformed the lives of millions of persons. If cataracts, the commonest cause for eye surgery, are your complaint, and your doctor has recommended eye surgery, by means of it you may have your vision restored, but here, too, let me advise caution. All cataract surgery is not needed.

Ophthalmology, the oldest surgical specialty, has in the last couple of decades brought forth remarkable innovations and modifications of old methods that make its surgeries easier to bear. The specialty is astir with new ideas. All to the good, but in some instances you may find it difficult to know whether you should accept an exciting new operation now or wait for the next improvement that is sure to come along. Let's see what we can find out.

CATARACT SURGERY

One ophthalmologist has said, "Cataract surgery today is safer than tonsillectomy." An unfortunate comparison. Although tonsillectomy may rarely threaten life, it's useless. Cataract surgery, as a rule, is useful.

Popular too: about a million operations a year to fill a growing need as our population ages ("Cataracts," 1987). Seventy-five percent of Americans sixty-five or older, we are told, will develop cataracts. Many with this disease don't lose significant vision, but estimates are that cataracts do disable 5 to 10 million individuals each year in the United States. People who refuse cataract surgery make up a large part of our blind population, says Frank Newell (1982), a Chicago ophthalmologist.

HISTORY

Introduced by the glass workers of Venice, spectacles first made their appearance about 1270. Not until 1753, however, did Jacques Daviel of Paris describe a method to extract a cataract that was not significantly modified until the middle of the nineteenth century, when Albrecht Von Graefe of Berlin improved the technique and thereby helped to establish the specialty of ophthalmology (Clendening, 1942).

Incidentally, an ophthalmologist is an M.D. who has taken special training to treat eye diseases and perform eye surgery. An optometrist, whose designation is confusingly similar, is not an M.D., but he has had special training to test vision, prescribe eyeglasses or eye exercises, fit contact lenses, and screen patients for eye diseases. The optometrist is expected to refer patients with eye diseases to an ophthalmologist. An optician (still another op- name) fills the prescriptions for glasses and contact lenses written by an ophthalmologist or an optometrist.

By 1910 the British ophthalmologist, Lt. Colonel Henry Smith, had done 24,000 cataract extractions in his Indian clinics (cataracts are more prevalent in India than in Europe and perhaps more prevalent in our Sun Belt than in the northern part of the country), and he instructed ophthalmologists from all over the world in his methods (Garrison, 1929). The operation was accepted as safe and effective; it became relatively stable technically. During the last fifteen years, however, it has been modified considerably, especially with the introduction, or reintroduction, of the intraocular lens (IOL) implant. Most ophthalmologists now insert an IOL to replace the cataract, thereby doing away with thick, coke-bottle-bottom spectacles or contact lenses after surgery.

NATURE OF THE DISEASE

The normal lens is a crystal-clear, flexible, egg-shaped structure about an eighth of an inch thick—convex on both front and back and enclosed in a transparent capsule. It has no nerve supply, and lacking a blood supply as well, it gets its nourishment from the liquid that surrounds it. The lens focuses light rays that pass through the pupil onto the light-sensitive retina at the back of the eye. Located just behind the iris, the lens is held by muscles attached around its edge, which will contract to flatten the lens when the eye focuses on distant objects or relax to thicken it when viewing near objects.

In midlife the lens becomes stiff, no longer thickening when the muscles relax, and because of that, reading glasses are required to focus on near objects. Sometime later, usually after fifty, the lens protein begins to denature (in the way the white of an egg becomes denatured and opaque when heated), and we have the beginning of a "senile" cataract. The lens gradually turns yellow and cloudy to the point where its diminished transparency blurs the vision; halos appear around lights at night. An almost inevitable process of aging, perhaps senile cataracts should not, strictly speaking, be called a disease. In any case, the ophthalmologist may not be able to draw a hard and fast line between an eye that has a cataract and an aging eye that does not.

Among causes of cataracts other than aging, some of which may bring it on early, are chemical or mechanical injuries, diabetes, parathyroidism (a glandular condition that causes low blood calcium), German measles during pregnancy (resulting in infant cataract), radiation, and electrical shock. Congenital cataracts, which are present at birth, may be inherited, but senile cataracts are not.

If you have cataracts, you may have noted as an early visual change a decrease in farsightedness ("second sight"), or if you are nearsighted, an increase in your nearsightedness, which may be temporarily corrected by new glasses. Other symptoms: improved vision in dim light, the sensation of a film on the eye, fuzzy vision, blurry vision, and difficulty in night vision because of halos or scattered lights. As the cataract matures, it becomes visible through the pupil, which then appears grayish rather than black.

Although his regular examinations are refined by many complex instruments, the ophthalmologist can make the diagnosis of cataract using nothing more than his ophthalmoscope (the flashlight-sized, hand-held instrument with which he peers into your eye). Its view of the retina will be partially blocked by the cataract.

You'll need surgery when your cataract-impaired vision interferes with your normal activities, something that varies from person to person. Someone with a job or a hobby that requires acute vision will opt for surgery sooner than someone whose life requires less demanding sight. "There's generally no reason to rush into surgery," says Dr. Jerome Bettman, who heads the ethics committee of the American Academy of Ophthalmology ("Cataracts," 1987). "It usually doesn't matter whether a cataract is removed early or late." The mere presence of a cataract is not an indication for surgery. Sometimes years pass before cataracts interfere seriously with vision.

Because it adds risk, insertion of an intraocular lens at the time of cataract extraction may be omitted in certain patients: those who have only one eye; those who have severe myopia of over 7 diopters (a measure of refractive power)—retinal detachment is the concern here; and those who have had a poor operative result in the fellow eye.

THE OPERATION

Under regional anesthesia, usually, the ophthalmologist makes a small incision at the edge of the cornea, a bit of the iris is removed at its rim, and the lens is extracted with the help of enzymes and various delicate sucking and freezing probes. Either the entire lens is removed, including its capsule (intracapsular extraction), or the lens and the anterior capsule are removed with retention of the posterior capsule (extracapsular extraction). The extracapsular extraction has become the favored choice because the posterior lens capsule then remains to serve as support for the intraocular lens implant.

Ambulatory surgery with extracapsular extraction and an intraocular implant (IOL), now the favored operation (Dowling and Bahr, 1985), has replaced what fifteen years ago was an intracapsular extraction followed by a two- to four-day hospital stay. Before IOL came to dominate the field, surgery left you with no lens (aphakia) and very blurry vision until you could be fitted with thick cataract spectacles or contact lenses. Now, with an IOL to replace the clouded cataract lens immediately, you rise from the operating table with clear distant vision. Because the eye muscles which normally change the thickness of the lens cannot change the thickness of the IOL for near adaption, you'll need reading spectacles.

The IOL is usually placed behind the iris in the posterior chamber—the normal position of the original lens. The refractive power required of the IOL, and thus its precise shape, is determined by measuring the refractive power of the cornea with a special instrument and the length of the eye with an ultrasonography instrument.

The current popularity of IOLs came about without the support of controlled clinical tests to compare their use with simple extraction and contact lenses; no clinical tests are planned. Comparison would be difficult, and at this time pointless, because the technique and the kinds of IOLs used change rapidly. As IOLs are much easier to live with than cataract spectacles or contact lenses, they have simply taken over. In time some of the IOLs will probably slip out of position or otherwise fail—no prosthesis lasts forever—but no one expects their use to be abandoned.

Complications occur, usually due to damage of the cornea. Altogether, however, few patients suffer serious, sight-threatening complications. Perhaps one patient in 10,000 suffers complications such as hemorrhage or infection, which may result in total loss of vision. Less than 5 percent of patients experience any complications. Detachment of the retina, one of the complications, requires corrective surgery.

Over 90 percent of patients have better vision after cataract surgery, and objective measurements of function and mental status in elderly patients show improvement too. Someone needing the operation shouldn't be denied it on the basis of age (Applegate et al., 1987).

ALTERNATIVES

If you have an early cataract, new glasses, as an alternative to surgery, may improve your vision, but no medical treatment will clear the opaque lens. Eye exercises won't improve your vision nor will diet. If cataracts seriously impair your vision, there is no satisfactory alternative to surgical extraction of the cataract.

Some ophthalmologists have carried the idea of lens removal farther by removing the clear lens and replacing it with an IOL for severe nearsightedness. Not generally recommended, however (see below).

REFRACTIVE SURGERY—FOR NEARSIGHTEDNESS OR FARSIGHTEDNESS

RADIAL KERATOTOMY

For the many nearsighted people who believe that their beauty or convenience is sacrificed by wearing glasses or contact lenses, eye surgery now, tentatively, offers radial keratotomy, epikeratophakia, or IOLs as alternatives. (Ophthalmologists employ many big words in a tradition that attempts to bridge languages and provide a shorthand for what might be a lengthy description in simpler words. They may also attempt to make these operations seem more mysterious that they really are. Healers, from shamans to ophthalmologists, have always been strong on mumbo jumbo.) I'll try to describe these eye operations simply, but remember, they are still experimental—don't accept any of them carelessly.

In the nearsighted eye the lens focuses the distant image in front of the retina; the eyeball is too long for its lens system. In the operation called radial keratotomy, the surgeon, by making radial incisions that begin just outside the pupil and run out to the edge of the cornea (the transparent part of the eye), intends to make the cornea bulge a little near the edge and thus become flatter in the central part to reduce its refractive index. When successful this corrects the myopia. At first ophthalmologists used as many as twenty-four to thirty-two radial incisions (none penetrating the cornea), but now they believe four, six, or eight incisions to be as effective.

Potentially blinding complications have been uncommon but possible (Goldsmith, 1985), and the operation has been plagued by uncertain results and lesser complications. The corneal scarring may cause glare and make it hard to tolerate contact lenses should they be needed. Small abscesses in the incisions may produce excessive scarring.

Those skilled with the technique claim that they can correct 4 to 5 diopters of myopia (quite severe nearsightedness) with a fair degree of predictability, but poor predictability and variable results have been the major problems (Binder, 1984). A multicenter study, the Prospective Evaluation of Radial Keratotomy (PERK), in their three-year followup of 410 patients, found that 57 percent remained corrected to within one diopter of correct refraction, but 27 percent remained uncorrected, though there may have been some improvement, and 16 percent were overcorrected (Kirn, 1987a). This is not good enough.

G. O. Waring III, director of the PERK study, says, "We all know it can work. We're just not sure how to fine-tune it to make it work precisely. We continue to look for ways to control the surgery better . . ." The PERK study will continue until 1990. (See Chapter 18 for a description of a legal battle growing out of this study.) Jerome Bettman, spokesman for the American Academy of Ophthalmology, says: "There is evidence to suggest that the incidence of RK [the operation] is decreasing." Most ophthalmologists intend to wait for more confirmation. Shouldn't you wait too?

REBUILDING THE CORNEA, EPIKERATOPHAKIA

Rather than merely make the little incisions of a radial keratotomy, ophthalmologists are now reshaping the cornea in order to correct nearsightedness (Kirn, 1987b). In an operation called keratomileusis, a slice from the top of the cornea is actually removed, frozen, and lathed to change its shape; the modified disk of cornea is then stitched back into place. Sounds risky—too easy to make an irreversible mistake.

This operation grew into something called epikeratoplasty or epikeratophakia (less risky, its advocates say). The cornea is not removed, just scraped a bit, and then a disk-shaped, donor corneal graft of precisely the correct shape is stitched in place over it. By this means the anterior (front) surface of the cornea is flattened, thus correcting the myopia. The operation has also been used for refractive defects such as lens absence in children and for the recontouring and reinforcing of the cornea in a disease called keratoconus. A nationwide clinical study has reported favorably on its use in 313 patients with myopia (McDonald et al., 1987). Advantages include a lack of vision-threatening complications and no danger of rejection; disadvantages: lack of stability and predictability. Dr. Waring, whom I quoted with respect to radial keratotomy, says that refinement of the technique is required before surgeons will be able to achieve ideal results. Don't let anyone "refine the technique" on your corneas.

REPLACEMENT OF A HEALTHY LENS WITH AN IOL TO CORRECT MYOPIA

Lens removal is another alternative in this line of aggressive surgeries that may save the cosmetically sensitive or those with specially demanding jobs from the embarrassment and inconvenience of spectacles or contact lenses. As in the cataract operation, this operation replaces the lens with a plastic substitute, but now the surgeon is extracting a *healthy* lens! The plastic lens, inserted in the eye itself, provides the correction. Hardly a sensible plan for a young client, because any foreign body has an uncertain and limited lifespan. Furthermore, a plastic lens lacks the flexibility of a normal lens, and therefore cannot adapt for near vision. Reading glasses are required. In addition, the risk of retinal detachment is high, say critics. A prospective clinical study is in the works, but this operation may lose out to epikeratophakia before the study's completion.

Wait. Wear your glasses, or if you have an important date, squint a little when you need to find your way.

FARSIGHTEDNESS—RADIAL THERMOCOAGULATION

Svyatoslav Fyodorov, the same ophthalmologist who introduced radial keratotomy, has now proposed radial thermocoagulation to correct far-sightedness. He hails, by the way, from the Soviet Union, unexpected origin for an imaginative new vanity surgery—which may, of course, still find its largest natural market in Southern California.

To correct farsightedness the curvature of the cornea must be increased rather than flattened, as in radial keratotomy. A small metal probe inserted into the cornea for 0.3 seconds and heated to 600 degrees Centigrade does the job. The microscopic burn so produced increases the curvature of the central cornea, causing the light rays to be focused exactly on the retina. In addition to treating farsightedness, the operation has been used to fine-tune radial keratotomy cases where there has been an overcorrection (Shader, 1987).

If these schemes work out, surgery for nearsightedness, farsightedness, or astigmatism might be sold to one third of the population—at, let us say, one-k bucks per eye, big business, billions. Most ophthalmologists, cautious by nature, remain cautious, however; and I think you should remain cautious too. As I noted above, ophthalmologists have undertaken a multicenter study of radial keratotomy, PERK, that has already shed some light, but it stirred up a legal battle (described in Chapter 18) that dragged the whole issue of clinical trials into murky waters (Norman, 1985; Duffey, 1988–89). The rather audacious enterprise of medical scientists to propel clinical medicine into the scientific age by way of clinical tests was threatened. The court's decision favored the directors of the PERK study, but legal procedure may again interrupt the course of scientific inquiry.

16

Cancer Surgery

Surgery and its partners, chemotherapy and radiation, cure nearly half of all cancers. Among the major cancers, surgery alone is able to cure cases of colon, lung, breast, uterine, and prostate cancer. It can cure several less common cancers. If in desperation you have considered a trip to Mexico for laetrile, a bout with the macrobiotic diet, or imaging to tune up your immune system—all notoriously inept therapies—consider surgery first; it may be your best hope. Oncologists (who provide chemotherapy) and radiotherapists now play a bigger role than they once did, but for most cancers they work with the surgeon rather than as alternative therapists. The cancer at its primary location has to be removed; that's the surgeon's job.

Is some cancer surgery unnecessary? If in the long run surgery fails to cure, it may in some sense—perhaps an economic sense—have been of little use. But it's certainly not unnecessary in the way that a tonsillectomy or a cesarean section is often unnecessary. No intervention at all or a medical intervention is usually better than those operations, but for cancer there may be no reasonable alternative to surgery. Although too often the expectation of surgical cure may end in disappointment, a recommendation of surgery for cancer is a signal of hope. You have a chance of cure, maybe a very good one.

Thus, the decision to have an operation becomes straightforward if not easy. In the best circumstances you accept the operation with an honest estimate of your chances. Because there are borderline cases, however, and because cancer overtreatment has been common—both by surgeons and oncologists—you may want to know something about the record of cancer surgery, about the nature of this complex, intractable disease: its causes, its alternative treatments, and its prevention.

Challenged a few decades ago by an apparent need, surgeons learned to take out more and more organs and structures. Blood transfusions, an improved comprehension of the physiology of trauma, and safer anesthesia made big operations possible. Investigators measured the responses of the body to surgery, and learned how to reinforce or alter them to provide better care during and following surgery. Surgical mortality rates fell. Due to an uncertain balance, at the time, between possible achievement and actual need, however, they didn't really know how much anatomy they ought to excise.

Enthusiastic by nature and aroused by the potential of their new technical competence, they floundered around in the surgical swamplands of total gastrectomy (all the stomach), cerebral hemispherectomy (half the brain), superradical mastectomy (the breast plus the accessible lymph nodes within and without the chest and other nearby tissues), four-quarter amputation (one-quarter of the body frame), and even hemicorporectomy (half the body!—about as far as you can go). They could do these things; their patients survived. Did their surgical gymnastics work?

Carmen T., a fifty-six-year-old woman who had noticed blood in her stools, was found to have a cancer of the large intestine. When it was resected (surgically removed), cancer was found in adjacent lymph nodes, which were also resected. Then, as part of a plan to resect these spreading cancers more aggressively (second-look operations), though she had no symptoms, she was operated upon a second time in six months. More lymph nodes, now with identifiable cancer, were excised. Similar operations were repeated every few months; each time the surgeon excised any cancer that had by then appeared. Cancerous nodules were removed from her liver and from her lung. She survived eight of these second-look operations before the effort was finally abandoned without achieving a cure.

I did some of those eight operations myself. To me, and others, the project seemed reasonable at the time. How else were we going to get rid of *all* the tumor (a requirement for cure) except by removing the tumor wherever it appeared? X ray couldn't cure that kind of cancer; it still can't: Chemotherapy wasn't available; now that it is available, it doesn't cure that kind of cancer either. Surgery was all we had, but it wasn't enough.

OVERTREATMENT?

It took a while for a surgical consensus to turn away from these big or repeated operations. The consensus isn't complete: Surgeons still perform second-look operations, and Tom Starzl, of Pittsburgh, has replaced cancerous, intra-abdominal organs, including the liver, pancreas, duodenum, stomach, spleen and some of the colon, en masse, at one operation, with a large "organ cluster" transplantation. This quite rightly has been described by a colleague as an "impressive surgical feat." One patient has survived six months (Goldsmith, 1989). It is too early to tell if this new kind of aggressive cancer surgery will affect survival, but, as in the past, it may turn out that cancer doesn't tend to contain itself within any neat surgical boundaries.

Convincing evidence to define the limitations of cancer surgery have appeared for breast cancer (Chapter 9). Surgeons had used the radical mastectomy (in which the entire breast, chest wall muscles, and lymph nodes of the armpit were removed) since the last decade of the nineteenth century. Assuming that cancer advanced in orderly stages from a local to a regional and then to a general disease, they took out the nearby tissues and the nodes to which the cancer might have made its first, as yet undetected, advance in the early stages of the disease. Only in the last couple of decades, after eighty years with the radical operation, have surgeons, using controlled clinical studies, learned that the radical mastectomy went too far. Breast cancer didn't behave quite the way they thought it did.

No other major cancers have been subjected to controlled studies similar to those for breast cancer, but the breast cancer findings support a way of viewing other cancers that plays down aggressive surgery's role. It seems that the nature of the cancer—is it local or general?—and the amount of spread at the time of surgery are far more decisive in predicting outcome than the character and extent of the operation. If it is a local disease, local excision will cure. But if there has been clinical spread, even though the spread might appear to be removable, the cancer may be a different kind of disease, a general disease.

In compliance with this concept, doctors may regard surgery as unavailing for the general disease. In practice, however, when there's no other hope, except possibly chemotherapy, why not do something? Try surgery anyway. Who will complain? Overtreatment for some cancers thereby becomes common. Frequent examples are found among cancers of the lung, rectum, pancreas, and thyroid (Crile, 1978).

Oncologists and radiotherapists overtreat too. Because their (often reluctantly made) recommendation of chemotherapy or X ray therapy may seem less momentous than the recommendation of a major operation, they may overtreat more frequently than do surgeons. These days most patients with incurable cancers lose their hair to chemotherapy before they lose their lives to cancer.

INCIDENCE

Cancer causes 22 percent of all deaths in the United States (second leading cause) for a total of more than 400,000 deaths a year (Smart, 1982). Twelve percent of men and 11 percent of women over seventy have at some time been given a diagnosis of cancer (Doll and Peto, 1981; Feldman et al., 1986). One in three Americans will have cancer and 1 in 5 dies of it. About 5 million persons now alive in the United States have at one time received a diagnosis of cancer. The most prevalent cancers overall are cancers of the lung, large intestine, breast, and prostate in that order, but among women breast cancer tops the list and among men prostatic cancer.

CAUSES

One hundred types of cancer are recognized, each considered by experts as a separate disease. But in all types the disease arises when some cell in the body starts to multiply without restraint and produces a family of descendants that invade the surrounding tissues and may be carried to distant parts by the blood or lymph. Thus, the crucial event in the origin of a cancer can be traced back to alterations of the founder cell.

Initiation and promotion stages in this process are regulated independently at different times by different agents. Initiation involves a brief and irreversible interaction between a cancer-causing agent and the genetic material of its target cell. This causes a mutation that transforms the target cell into an abnormal state in which its oncogenes become activated. These genes will direct cells to take up their abnormal, cancerous behavior. The initiation alone does not generate a clinically observable tumor (Weinberg, 1983).

As a second stage the cells must be acted on by a promoting agent. Though not mutagenic itself, the promoter, applied continuously, can cause transformed cells to proliferate and form a clinically evident cancer. As much as ten to twenty years of latency may occur between an initiation event and the appearance of a tumor.

Cigarette smoking, X rays, and certain chemicals are initiators (*Cancer Prevention*), but only a few relatively uncommon human cancers have been associated with clearly specific initiating (causative) agents: mesothelioma (cancer of the material lining various body cavities) of the lung with asbestos, for example, and Burkitt's lymphoma with the Epstein-Barr virus. Among major cancers, only lung cancer has been associated with a somewhat specific agent: inhaled tobacco smoke. For the other major cancers—breast, colon, prostate, pancreas, uterus, ovary—little is known of the initiating agents.

Promoting agents do not cause cancer by themselves, but they change cells already damaged by an initiator. Alcohol, for example, promotes the development of cancers in the mouth, throat, and possibly the liver when combined with an initiator, such as tobacco.

RISK FACTORS

An agent, either an initiator or a promoter, that has been linked to the cause of a particular cancer is called a risk factor. Contact with that agent increases an individual's risk of contracting that particular cancer. Of course, some risk factors, such as aging, are unavoidable, while others, known with various degrees of certainty, are avoidable—at least in principle: tobacco, radiation, alcohol, some components of diet and food additives, some features of occupational environment, and chemical carcinogens.

According to the National Cancer Institute, about 7,000 chemicals have been reported as having been tested for carcinogenicity in animals, and a little more than 1,500 of these have been reported to be carcinogenic (Maugh, 1978). Actual numbers may be smaller. The Delaney clause in the Food and Drug Act (a clause which prohibits the addition to processed foods of any compound that causes cancer in test animals) has fired a running debate concerning the reliability of projections from animal tests to human causation. It seems to be easier, in general, to cause cancer in an experimental animal than in man. Unfortunately, carcinogen-potency estimation is an inexact science, but it appears that any possible carcinogens in our food, added by farming or preservation methods, are much less important as risk factors than tobacco or a high fat intake.

RADIATION

Most of us receive our biggest lifetime dose of radiation, identified as a cause of cancer almost since it was first used in medicine, through X rays. Diagnostic X rays add up. Doctors have become sensitive to this danger, and modern techniques, such as xeromammography and the CAT scan, use commendably low radiation doses. Dentists use X ray less frequently than they once did. If nuclear power plants can be kept from leaking or exploding, they do not raise background radiation significantly. Long-term storage of perpetually dangerous waste may stand as the biggest power-plant-radiation problem. Nuclear warfare, though an overwhelming producer of radiation, would probably kill most of us before our radiation-induced cancers had time to sprout.

Low-level background radiation—now a worrisome issue through the discovery that radon may seep from the soil into many homes—remains an ill-defined risk. High radon levels, found in uranium mines, have been shown to cause lung cancer, and low concentrations have been assumed to increase the risk of cancer by an amount proportional to the dose, but some studies now challenge that assumption. One study found that lung cancer mortality was lower where radon exposure was high (Beardsley, 1988)! The Environmental Protection Agency's radon standards may be too strict and difficult to comply with. In any case, the general threat of background radiation appears to be relatively low compared to that of smoking or improper diet.

DIAGNOSTIC SCREENING PROGRAMS

Stimulated by the American Cancer Society, the National Institutes of Health, and the many voluntary supporters of various screening projects, doctors have for fifty years tried to improve their cure rate by means of early cancer detection. They plead with us to have regular checkups; they establish cancer detection centers; they teach us in public campaigns how to examine ourselves in order to detect "early signs," thus conspicuously nourishing our hypochondriacal inclinations (and simultaneously discovering some small cancers, I must add). If, as described above, the disease starts in a single cell, which multiplies unrestricted to become a local tumor before it spreads to become uncurable, we should try to detect small, local cancers. Remove them surgically then, for cures.

That's the sensible plan, but like any simple medical plan, this plan encounters the complexities of biological reality. Cancer, we discover, is complex and various. In some of its varieties, it may spread even before the original tumor can be detected by our most sensitive methods. With such cases the best "early diagnosis" we can make wouldn't help. With other varieties, at the opposite end of a malignancy range, spread may never occur during the victim's lifetime. Though an "early diagnosis" of such varieties can be made, it really wouldn't be responsible for the favorable outcome. In such a case, you might even conclude that "cancer" was the wrong diagnosis.

How could one make the right diagnosis? A "cancer" should be a potentially lethal disease. Therefore, if diagnosis was the only concern, you could simply wait to see if the disease was ultimately lethal—a useless and morally intolerable plan. We need an earlier diagnosis, so the diagnosis is made by a pathologist who looks at a microscopic slide of the tumor and then declares it to be a cancer or not—a matter of training and skill. Unintentionally, perhaps, pathologists assume a godlike role.

Supported by the considerable experience of their venerable profession, they have learned to do very well, but I think that they are inclined, when in doubt, to overdiagnose a little. If they say something is benign and later it spreads to kill, they have made a grave error. The patient, treated as the carrier of a benign lesion, has lost his chance for cure. If, on the other hand, the pathologist labels something as cancer and the patient is "cured" of something that really wasn't a potentially spreading, lethal cancer, the pathologist escapes criticism, and medical science, or an "alternative" or quack therapy if it were used, may get undeserved credit. The error may not even be recognized, but if it is, and the pathologist wants to achieve technical accuracy, all he has to do is review the microscopic slides and declare that, because of some details not readily apparent at the first examination, the tumor was not a cancer after all. Or the pathologist may simply agree with the pleased surgeon, who excised the tumor, by stating that the surgeon's operation was marvelously effective after all. No one will complain of that outcome.

Early detection schemes have worked best for breast cancer. Perhaps a fourth of the total mortality due to breast cancer might be prevented by examining women over fifty every one to three years (Cairns, 1985). Though by now Pap smears have been applied one or more times to at least 75 percent of adult women in the United States, lack of adequately controlled studies has prevented precise determination of their benefits for treating cancer of the uterus. Screening programs for cancer of the skin and mouth *have* proved effective, partly because these sites are easily accessible. Regrettably, no great benefit has come from detecting lung cancer by chest X ray prior to symptoms. By the time it is detected, it has spread. In summary, early-diagnosis screening programs sometimes bring benefits, sometimes not. Aside from questions of efficacy, however, it appears unlikely that the United States or any country will ever be able to afford the cost of testing the majority of its population annually for the earliest signs of each of the major cancers.

DIAGNOSTIC METHODS. STAGING.

Preoperative diagnosis has become so complex and expensive that you may wonder if all the tests are necessary. Probably not. A lot of time, trouble, and delay may precede your operation. Each diagnostic technique has its own set of complications, and if the results are indefinite, the test may have to be repeated or supplemented. Why not skip all of them—just go ahead with the operation? The surgeon could at least take a look, then if possible do something.

Once a common strategy during a time of "exploratory laparotomies," this direct, surgical mode has been abandoned to diagnostic specialists who use CAT scans, NMR (nuclear magnetic resonance), ultrasound, xeromammography, fine-needle biopsies, and various "staging" methods before resorting, finally, to a surgical exploration. As each new diagnostic technique has appeared, its availability alone has encouraged its use. Something new becomes interesting, even exciting, and if the machinery sits there waiting (and still to be paid for), why not use it?

By using this expensive diagnostic apparatus your doctors may plan the course of your management logically with very small risk to you. They obtain marvelous internal views with a cat scan and with NMR—new perspectives with far more detail than previous X rays ever revealed. Used with needle biopsies, these techniques may provide a definitive diagnosis preoperatively in tumors that were previously accessible, and finally identifiable, only by major surgery. Then, with an accurate diagnosis in hand they may devise treatment that may include chemotherapy, x-ray therapy, or even delay, as well as surgery. The champions of these techniques find sound clinical reasons for using everything available in almost every case. Something may be gained and very little lost—except money.

Money's lack may eventually slow their dissemination, but generous use of these new techniques is firmly based on a respected medical philosophy that places diagnosis before treatment. A wise doctor believes he ought to know what he is treating. At one time, approximately a century ago, when only a few specific treatments were available, clinical medicine began to achieve its modest scientific distinction by improving diagnosis—among leading doctors, diagnosis was the thing. The treatments they came up with might be only supportive—"symptomatic" they were called—remedies to keep the patient relatively comfortable while his body cured itself—if it could. Hot packs, aspirin, enemas, and reassurance were often all they had; they found little intellectual challenge in administering such nostrums. In contrast, diagnosis was an intellectual feat and an art that made medical practice a fascinating challenge. To most doctors, and probably to most of us if we think about it, it still makes good sense to seek a precise, accurate diagnosis before embarking on a possibly risky treatment course. Thus, users of these enormous, complex, modern, engineering miracles who seek an accurate diagnosis at low risk follow a sound and ancient tradition.

Doctors also use—and overuse—these diagnostic machines for personal legal protection. Don't skip anything along the way, they tell themselves, and then should the final result disappoint the client, you're a smaller malpractice target.

Cost, they say, will finally block this new technology's universal application. As health-care costs in the United States keep rising—by 9.8 percent in 1987 (L.A. Times, November, 19, 1988)—we learn that hospitals account for 39 percent of this enormous bill, and that hospitals attribute a considerable portion of their costs to this new technology. No one wants to turn away from technological excellence, yet there has been little solid evidence that it significantly improves our chances of surviving most cancers. In a tight economy, where political interest in curbing health-care expenses grows, this may become evidence for holding back.

THE OPERATION

The surgeon intends to remove all of the cancer with minimal mutilation—a clear objective but one hard to achieve in ideal balance. With some cancers, the common cancer of the skin, for example, he has merely to excise the growth with a reasonable margin of normal tissue. With other cancers—a cancer of the stomach that has spread to the liver or the lung, say—any operation will fail to cure. He is unable to achieve his ideal objective, but he may still remove the diseased stomach in order to relieve symptoms temporarily—palliative surgery.

With many major cancers—breast cancer or colon (large intestine) cancer—for example, the disease may have reached adjacent lymph nodes when first diagnosed, in a spread not evident to the surgeon, but detectable by the pathologist when he examines the many nodes in the surgical specimen. Although the surgeon can't be sure how far the disease has extended at the time of surgery, he takes out areas of potential lymph-node spread because he believes that he will in some cases obtain a cure not possible by lesser surgery.

This concept, central to cancer surgery for decades, has been sorely tried by the controlled studies of breast cancer (Chapter 9). Limited surgery for apparently limited disease, supplemented, it is true, by X ray and sometimes by chemotherapy, has proved to be effective. Breast cancer (seemingly) and other cancers (possibly) appear in various guises from the beginning—some widespread almost from the start, others local, perhaps for a long time. The results of surgical excision may depend more upon the nature of the cancer than on the range and nature of the surgery—provided, of course, that the primary tumor is adequately removed.

ADJUVANT OR ALTERNATIVE TREATMENTS

After discovering, early on, that surgery's record was far from ideal, therapists of various persuasions have been supplementing surgery or substituting for it with treatments ranging from the useless to the highly effective—one often about as popular as the other, at least for a while. Radiation, chemotherapy, and hormonal therapy, the most effective, will cure some cancers and suppress many all by themselves. Krebiozin and laetrile, two of the least effective, have raised false hopes and cured no one.

Hormonal therapy, which began in the 1890s, with the removal of the ovaries in hope of curing spreading breast cancer, finds use today for cancers of the breast, ovary, prostate, and testicle. Castration, its most definitive employment, may now be replaced by drugs to achieve similar effects—the estrogen inhibitor, tamoxifen, for example, acts as a substitute for oophorectomy (removal of the ovaries). Though hormonal therapy may impressively prolong a symptom-free life, cure with it is unusual.

As with hormonal therapy, radiation and chemotherapy have reached a complexity that results in reference texts as massive as those on surgery. I will attempt only a few summary comments. Both modalities achieve their effects by damaging cells. Radiation damages the immune system, the bone marrow, the lining of the intestines, and at the basic cellular level, it damages genetic material. When it works, it works because rapidly dividing cancer cells are more sensitive to radiation than are normal cells. With an easily accessible superficial cancer, such as a skin cancer, radiation cures. When the cancer is deep, the cancer must be destroyed without destroying too much normal tissue; this becomes possible, to a degree, with modern, high-powered machines carefully focused, that direct intense radiation where it is most needed. Some deep cancers— Hodgkins disease, cancer of the cervix of the uterus, and one kind of testicular cancer—can be effectively treated. Most deep cancers, however, cannot be cured by radiation.

About one fourth of all cancer patients take some form of chemotherapy during their initial hospital stay for cancer, and generally in the United States more than 200,000 patients receive chemotherapy each year. Yet benefits are established for only a low percentage of those treated (Cairns, 1985). Chemotherapy originated with the observation, dating back to WWI, that mustard gas damaged the bone marrow. Since then many reagents selectively injurious to cancer have been discovered, nearly all of which bind to DNA, causing damage that the cell cannot repair properly. Usually one agent is not enough. If all the cells in a cancer are to be destroyed, the therapist finds it necessary to use each chemical agent at the highest tolerable dose and to use different agents simultaneously.

Suitable subjects have benefited dramatically—those with childhood leukemia especially. Among childhood cancers two thirds of its victims appear to be cured or placed in prolonged, relapse free survival. Among adult cancers, choriocarcinoma (a rare cancer of the placenta) can now be cured at a saving of twenty to thirty lives a year. Combined radiation and chemotherapy treatment now cures most Hodgkin's disease victims. Results such as these have encouraged a large corps of oncologists and motivated thousands of patients to enlist in clinical trials. Nonetheless, John Cairns in a review article in *Scientific American* (1985) points out: "Apart from the success with Hodgkin's disease, childhood leukemia and a few other cancers, it is not possible to detect any sudden change in the death rates for any of the major cancers that could be credited to chemotherapy."

All told, adjuvant treatments now avert a few thousand (perhaps 2 or 3 percent) of the 400,000 yearly American cancer deaths. These are real gains, which might be increased a little without any new agents, but any further gains from wider use of current surgical or adjuvant therapy could not match the gains that might be achieved by prevention—by significant reduction or abolition of tobacco smoking, in particular.

INTERLEUKIN-2

Stimulating or suppressing the immune system as a form of cancer therapy (adoptive immunotherapy) has attracted attention and enough research energy to make interleukin-2 the new anticancer drug—but not quite a magic bullet, unfortunately (Rosenberg et al., 1987; Merz, 1986). Possibly immunotherapy will be the way to go. One authority says that "we may be near the end of our search for a meaningful direction in the immunotherapy of cancer" (Durant, 1987). A few early results have been impressive, but the treatment is toxic, and no one claims that it is ready for widespread use.

THE FRINGE. LAETRILE, MACROBIOTIC DIET, ETC.

When surgery and conventional adjuvant therapy have failed to cure, or even before their failure becomes evident, desperation may conquer reason in anyone afflicted with this hateful disease. Try anything, what's to lose? Nostrums such as Krebiozin, a drug of twenty years past little remembered now, and laetrile, more recently the objective of Mexican pilgrimages, both supported only by anecdotes and no solid evidence at all, reach a popularity that temporarily exceeds the attractions of Lourdes or TV faith healers. As in the past, a fraudulent industry may quickly build on the futile hopes of the stricken.

A doctor whose prostatic cancer has shown impressive remission after castration, as it sometimes does, attributes his improvement to diet rather than to the conventional treatment. He writes a book, and many otherwise rational people try, as best they can, to follow a stringent, mystically derived "macrobiotic diet" (Sattilaro, 1982). Or they practice "imaging," though no good evidence has been presented to show that imaging improves the immune response to cancer, as supposed, or that it has had any objective effect on cancer (Simonton et al., 1978). Pilgrimages are made to the Philippines where "psychic surgeons," who are merely sleight-of-hand tricksters, claim to remove tumors without surgical incision. A book entitled *Love, Medicine & Miracles* (Siegel, 1986) concerned with the issues of living and dying with cancer, and with the hope of recovery through self-help, perhaps in the company of others afflicted, becomes a best-seller.

Traditional medicine, by so often failing with this disease, provides plenty of space for cults and "alternative" treatments. The traditional doctor, attentive to his difficult and scientific quest for a real, objective cure (a "five-year survival"), may be so exhausted and despairing over his failure that he seems to abandon his desperate patient. The patient doesn't give up as quickly and finds support wherever he can. With plans such as the hospice movement, some parts of traditional medical practice have responded to the patient's need, but many patients want to search further. They seek encouragement and prefer false promises to none at all. Surely, traditional medicine's accusation that "alternative" methods lack scientific validity is an inadequate response. Afflicted persons need help; they need help for a graceful way of dying. A cure for cancer won't eliminate this need.

SPONTANEOUS RECOVERY

Does cancer ever disappear by itself? Yes, but very rarely. Tildon Everson and Warren Cole (1966), who studied 176 reported cases of spontaneous recovery, estimated that the rate of spontaneous recovery is probably from 1 in 10,000 to 1 in 100,000.

RESULTS

How are we doing in the War Against Cancer? If we could put a man on the moon, the argument once went, we could surely muster enough resources to lick cancer. There have been a few striking improvements and many small benefits, but according to John C. Bailar III and Elaine M. Smith of the Harvard School of Public Health (1986), "We are losing the war against cancer, notwithstanding progress against several uncommon forms of the disease, improvements in palliation, and extension of the productive years of life." They base their conclusion on change in the age-adjusted mortality rate of all cancers combined in the total population. Their comments in no way argue against seeking the earliest possible diagnosis and the best possible management of cancer, but their main conclusion states: "Some 35 years of intense effort focused largely on improving treatment must be judged a qualified failure . . . A shift in research emphasis, from research on treatment to research on prevention, seems necessary . . ."

As might be expected, the National Cancer Institute, which in its own best interests has been reporting improvement regularly over the years, disagrees (Culliton, 1987). Cancer patients are living longer, the institute says. In rebuttal to this claim, the General Accounting Office joins the fray by pointing out that cancer patients aren't living longer; they are just known to have cancer for a longer time before they die (Merz, 1987). No matter what conclusions are reached concerning general success or failure, everyone supports Bailar and Smith's emphasis on prevention.

PREVENTION

In principle the approximately 90 percent of United States cancers that may be environmentally determined are preventable. Yet, except for tobacco, few specific agents have been pinpointed.

Eliminate the initiator and the promoting agents, described above under "Causes," and encourage the consumption of or exposure to antipromoting agents—if such various agents can be identified.

With the identification we now have, the best strategy requires abolition of smoking—the most prevalent promoting or initiating agent of lung and several other cancers. As much as 85 percent of smoking-related cancers could be prevented (Smart, 1982), but results still lag far behind that estimate. Critics of national policy point out that the Federal government subsidizes the tobacco industry and fails to raise strong inducements to stop smoking. Why? Smoking, the critics say, saves the government about $35,000 in Social Security payments per smoker, because smokers die younger than nonsmokers!

Second only to cigarette smoking, diet as a cause became evident because of large differences in cancer incidence that could not be attributed to the genes. Second generation Japanese in this country, for example, have a cancer-incidence pattern similar to that of other Americans rather than the pattern found among relatives they left behind in Japan. After they live here and eat our food, they acquire our cancers. Doll and Peto estimate that 35 percent (possible range: 10–70 percent) of American cancers may be caused by diet (1981), with dietary fat most clearly established as a promoter. From this comes the recommendation to reduce our fat consumption to 30 percent or less of total calories.

Possible antipromoters, whose consumption reduces the likelihood of contracting cancer, include dietary fiber, vitamins A,C, and E, the trace element selenium, and certain compounds found in vegetables such as broccoli, cabbage, and cauliflower (Willett and MacMahon, 1984). Dietary elements doubtless have both important causative and protective roles, but despite the work of epidemiologists and the confident enthusiasm of health-food promoters, information about specific dietary factors remains generally inconsistent or incomplete. Hence, special committees on general dietary reform have made rather conservative and often controversial recommendations. The National Research Council has offered two lists of recommendations, one in 1980 and one in 1982, both attacked by critics. The National Academy of Sciences, with a 1,000-page report, a council on Agricultural Science and Technology, the American Cancer Society, and the National Institutes of Health, as well as countless less prestigious, but often more spirited, authorities have gotten into the action.

General recommendations of the National Institutes of Health (which include more than diet) are these: Don't smoke. Eat foods high in fiber, low in fat (30 percent or less fat). Eat fresh fruits and vegetables. Avoid too much sunlight, avoid unnecessary X rays, drink alcohol only in moderation. Take estrogens only as long as necessary (*Cancer Prevention*). The National Research Council's second recommendation list (Maugh, 1982; Pariza, 1984) is similar to these recommendations, though the NRC didn't advise an increased fiber intake. However, they did advise reduced consumption of cured, pickled, and smoked foods. Other authorities have advised an increased consumption of complex carbohydrates, such as grains, fruits, and vegetables, and a decreased consumption of simple carbohydrates, such as refined sugars. The NAS, the NIH, and the NRC have not recommended supplementary vitamins or minerals for cancer prevention, because fresh fruits and vegetables, which they do recommend, provide enough. Although I don't think the evidence justifies the trouble and expense of taking all the supplementary vitamin and mineral pills that are being consumed, they are relatively harmless. If you crave them, take them. Sir William Osler, famous early twentieth-century physician, antedating the present craving, said, "The desire to take medicine is perhaps the greatest feature which distinguishes man from the animals."

To the distress of some critics, the official sources I have quoted lie low regarding artificial food additives—not enough evidence, they say. Nor do they say much about the risk of cancer you may incur at work—hold off until we know more. Conservative by their responsibility and their nature, they are bound to be cautious in their recommendations—and to modify them, no doubt, as more evidence appears.

SURGICALLY TREATED CANCERS NOT DESCRIBED IN OTHER CHAPTERS

Lung cancer, our most frequent major cancer, has a rising incidence in most parts of the world. Among white males it increased at annual rates of up to 10 percent during the 1970s, slowed, then decreased a little for 1982 and 1983; during recent years, it has increased for females. Accounting for 15 percent of all invasive cancers in the United States, it killed 130,000 persons in 1986 (Feldman et al., 1986). Surgical resection cures more than half of those who have resectable tumors without lymph-node spread (Mayer and Patterson, 1988), but unfortunately, limited disease is not the usual finding, and we achieve a combined five-year survival of only 8 percent for men and 12 percent for women (Gunby, 1980). Chest surgery is indicated for approximately half, and among these resection for cure is possible in half. Radiotherapy reduces local recurrence rate after resection of the commonest type, but it does not increase survival rate. With small-cell carcinoma of the lung, a less common kind, however, addition of radiotherapy to combination chemotherapy has improved both response rates and survival (Perry et al., 1987).

Cancer of the colon and rectum, the second most common major cancer, shows an annual rise of 1 to 3 percent in Occidental countries; it causes 53,000 deaths a year in this country. Surgery, which may improve life even when it doesn't cure, provides the only acceptable curative treatment. Survival following surgery is reduced by half when the lymph nodes are diseased. Stool tests for blood and examination of the entire inside of the bowel by a technique called colonoscopy have enhanced diagnosis and improved outlook for persons in whom polyps, possibly precancerous, are found.

Good news! Cancer of the stomach, once our most common cancer, and a cancer difficult to cure (10 percent alive at five years), has, on a happy note, been decreasing in all parts of the world (Gunby, 1980). Its incidence has dropped five-fold in the United States during the past fifty years—a surprising fact, not attributable to medical effort, but nonetheless a most encouraging development on the cancer scene. We must have been doing something right—but exactly what? Conjectures abound, and the most popular of these attribute the decline to changes in our diet—less smoked and pickled food, less nitrates, more raw vegetables, changes in food preservation methods. Though stomach cancer's lower incidence was not the result of research or planning, its fact supports proper food and proper living as the best way to prevent cancer.

Although thyroid cancer, the most common of endocrine cancers, in several parts of the developing world is still the most common cancer in females (female incidence generally exceeds that in males by a 3 to 1 ratio), its incidence is decreasing in the United States, where, by the way, it was once caused by unnecessary radiotherapy and then overtreated for many years with radical removal of the entire thyroid gland (Crile, 1978).

The liver, often a site of spread for cancers that originated elsewhere (metastases), also experiences a primary cancer. Caused by alcoholism, hepatitis B virus, exposure to vinyl chloride, use of oral contraceptives, injection of thorotrast (a dye once used for X rays), this cancer may be one of the most prevalent malignant diseases worldwide (Meyers, 1986). Only resection will prolong survival. If the tumor can be resected with no apparent remnant, an unusual event, five-year survival has ranged from 11 to 46 percent.

Gallbladder cancer, found three to four times as often in women as in men, has a surprisingly high incidence in American Indians. Most cases, 70 percent, have gallbladder stones. Surgery, the only successful treatment, usually fails to cure: only 4 percent survive five years.

Ovarian cancer, also a disease of gloomy prospect on the average, can be removed surgically in only about 20 percent of cases; the last twenty-five years have marked little improvement.

Glioblastoma, the most common cancer of the brain, is the most malignant of human neoplasms. Not all are glioblastomas; 15 percent of brain cancers are cancers of the lung, breast, skin (melanoma), or lymph nodes that have metastasized to the brain.

Pancreatic cancer, relatively infrequent, is increasing at 2 percent to 3 percent a year. Surgery, the only successful treatment, realizes a five-year survival rate in the United States of 1 percent.

Melanoma, the most malignant kind of skin cancer (5 percent of skin cancers), has shown a dramatic increase in Nordic countries. Perhaps more ultraviolet rays are getting through to these fair-skinned, and thus susceptible persons. Whites to blacks—20 to 1. Surgeons excise the tumor and a border of normal tissue and remove lymph nodes for diagnostic staging, or perhaps for treatment. Fifty percent long-term survival.

For oral cavity and tongue cancers—tobacco and alcohol the likely causes—surgeons use radical removal with reconstruction. Radiation and chemotherapy play a part, and five-year survival ranges from 15 to 25 percent for oral cavity, 40 percent for tongue. Lip cancer, a disease related to tobacco, sunlight exposure, and sex (87 percent male), can be cured by local excision or radiation if it hasn't spread. If it has, surgery removes the neck lymph-nodes as well.

Following are a few cancers for which surgery plays a part, but radiation or chemotherapy earns the credit for recent, dramatic improvement:

Testicular cancer, a disease of the young (age twenty to thirty-five), in its most prevalent form, seminoma, responds to radiation and chemotherapy as well as to surgical excision. Ninety percent five-year survival reported, and with recurrence, chemotherapy may bring about remissions in at least two thirds of cases (Weinerth, 1986).

Bone cancer among the old is usually the consequence of metastases from a primary tumor elsewhere, such as the breast or prostate. Primary cancer of the bone (osteosarcoma) appears in the young—mean age fifteen. Once treated by amputation with a 20 percent five-year survival, it is now treated with limb-preserving operations and adjunctive chemotherapy with a 50 percent, five-year, disease-free survival.

Surgery's role in Hodgkin's disease (a fatal disease of the lymph nodes, spleen, and lymphatic tissues) is an abdominal operation in which the surgeon removes the spleen and abdominal lymph nodes and takes a specimen of the liver. With this material, the pathologist and the oncologist determine the extent, the "stage," of the disease, information upon which the oncologist will plan the precise treatment. Combined radiation and chemotherapy now attain an 85 percent survival for Stages I and II (least advanced disease) and a 40–50 percent survival for Stage IV (most advanced and at one time uniformly fatal).

17
Protect the Young

TONSILLECTOMY AND ADENOIDECTOMY (T&A)

If your doctor has recommended a T&A for your child, take care; he may be simply adhering to a tradition, or to a "rite of passage" from infancy to childhood. As a child, he probably had a T&A himself, perhaps you did. But most likely your child doesn't need it—medically.

These operations were only rarely performed until a fantastic rise in popularity reached its peak in the 1930s when some 50 to 75 percent of all children, particularly those in the higher socioeconomic classes, were having their tonsils and adenoids removed (Fry, 1957). A 1943 study of New York children found that 94 percent of eleven-year-olds eventually had the operation. It was relatively easy—for the doc—and a good money maker; parents were willing; children did have fewer colds after the surgery—a consequence, in fact, of their growing up, not of the operation. Despite the lack of sound evidence to support its use for other than rare cases, about a million T&As a year were done in this country for many years.

Now after decades of opposition by medical scientists, after countless critical attacks in the medical and lay literature, and after a few controlled studies, its frequency has dropped to approximately that of a few other relatively overused operations, such as CABG and hysterectomy. About 280,000 were done in 1986.

As long ago as 1958 the president of the American Academy of Pediatricians, expressing the viewpoint of many physicians then, said, regarding the operation, "In the overwhelming majority of cases, it is useless" (Bakwin, 1958). Ten years later R. J. Haggerty, of the University of Rochester, said, "Today it is my impression that most academic pediatricians believe there are practically no indications for the removal of tonsils and adenoids." In 1976 Drs. Paradise and Bluestone of Pittsburgh, who were studying the operation scientifically with controlled clinical tests, wrote, "Most T&A's are done today for unproved medical indications." In a commentary Dr. Terrence S. Carden, Jr., said (1978), "If three quarters of a million young Americans were being subjected each year to a surgical procedure of doubtful benefit at a cost approaching $1 billion and untold cost in pain, suffering, and psychological trauma, the medical profession might expect a torrent of justifiable criticism." The profession has had some criticism, but probably not enough.

After being taught during medical school and my internship, in the late 1930s, that the operation had largely been discredited, I worked mostly in the somewhat protected environment of academic medicine for years and rarely saw a T&A on the operative schedule. If I thought about it at all, I thought that T&A had become an uncommon operation. But in 1975 a landmark report, *Surgery in the United States*, sponsored by the American College of Surgeons and the American Surgical Association, listed T&A as the *second* most frequent operation. Second? Bad enough, but the figures actually showed that T&A was *first*. It was the most common operation in the United States. The report, oddly, had listed normal vaginal delivery as first, calling it a more frequent surgical operation than T&A. Wait a minute! Is normal delivery a *surgical operation*? Or could the compilers of this report have placed normal delivery first in order to avoid some of the embarrassment of T&A? They were describing how their distinguished professional colleagues practiced medicine. Perhaps by this peculiar trick of definition, they diminished a little, at least in their own eyes, the preeminence in the surgical lineup of the tacky T&A.

T&A has been called an uncontrolled surgical experiment, a ritual, an enigma, more grandly a *pseudodoxia pediatrica*, more simply a problem, and finally an epidemic unchecked (the operation, that is, not the disease for which it is supposedly done).

THE NATURE OF TONSILS AND ADENOIDS

Tonsils and adenoids, the objects of the assault, are organs of the lymphatic system, a system which plays an essential role in the development and maintenance of immunity. They present a defensive barrier at the entrances of the digestive and respiratory tracts. Infectious agents invading this busy area are normally taken up by these organs, and in the process they become inflamed and enlarged. Even without infection, tonsils, adenoids, and all lymphatic organs are relatively large in small children; they shrink as we grow older.

When a small child has a head cold or a sore throat, the tonsils may appear enormous. Though the child is generally ill, the tonsils, especially if pointed out by an examiner, may be the most prominent sign of the illness. They appear to be the center of the trouble rather than merely part of the normal reaction to it.

As any parent knows, children have many respiratory infections. As the immune system strengthens over time, it will head off these infections, but if parents become exasperated while waiting, and the physician they consult feels that he has to do *something*, the child may lose his tonsils to surgery. Then, because the child improves, parents and doctor may conclude, in a simple logical error, that the strategy has "worked." But many things less painful and dangerous, including time alone, may "work." T&A has only a few sound indications.

INDICATIONS FOR T&A

Chronically recurring sore throats and head colds have been the commonest indications for recommending a T&A, but the operation has been used for about fifteen various, respiratory-infection-related complaints and a few remote, frivolous, or inappropriate complaints, such as learning difficulty or bed wetting.

Only a few relatively rare indications for the operation have been scientifically established. A type of heart failure caused by breathing obstruction has been dramatically relieved by the operation. Serious respiratory obstruction without heart failure stands as a sound indication. This and a type of weight loss resulting from obstruction to swallowing were the only categorical indications for T&A granted by a Workshop on Tonsillectomy and Adenoidectomy (1975).

As "reasonable" indications, not then established by adequate controlled studies, the workshop listed recurrent attacks of tonsillitis, nasal obstruction causing severe speech deformity, and recurrent, or chronic, middle ear infection—the latter two indications possibly requiring only adenoidectomy.

CONTROLLED STUDIES

More recently than that workshop, a controlled study, reported in 1984 by Paradise and Bluestone of Pittsburgh, compared T&A with medical treatment for children who might be considered to have the most persuasive, "reasonable" indications for surgery. Candidates had to have had at least seven documented episodes of throat infection in the previous year or three episodes per year for three years—a severity represented by less than 10 percent of the patients referred for tonsillectomy. Selected randomly, half the patients had a T&A, the other half were treated medically. In the first two years after entering the study, the surgical group did have fewer throat infections, but both groups improved, and by the third year the differences leveled out. The authors concluded that the results warranted the election of tonsillectomy for children meeting the trials' stringent eligibility criteria, but also that the results provided support for nonsurgical management of even those children.

The frequently commented-on overuse of T&A is apparently due to a stretching of these reasonable indications.

About 100 children a year die of the operation in the United States, usually of general anesthesia or hemorrhage. This is a low mortality rate, yet no one would recommend use of a new drug that killed 100 patients a year to treat a nonfatal, self-limited disease. Surgery deserves a similar assessment.

CURRENT STATUS

Perhaps the message is finally getting through; the rate of T&A (now at 280,000) has dropped to less than a third of its heyday, but that still discloses an amazing number of, mostly quiet, perpetrators. Those who do speak in support of the operation nowadays do so cautiously, claiming only that it is a good operation for the limited indications I have mentioned above. (To reach the current total those indications must be stretched.) Or they write about subsidiary issues such as how to make the process more efficient, whether or not the patient should be kept in hospital overnight following surgery. Postoperative hemorrhage, a significant risk, must be watched for, but in order to reduce costs the insurance companies want the patient sent home immediately.

Why has T&A remained so popular so long in the face of so much opposition and with so little evidence to justify it? I've read comments saying that the effectiveness of the operation has *not* been disproved. But I thought it was the other way around: Advocates of a therapy should *prove* the effectiveness of their method. Many practitioners must tend to ignore the research, or at least modify its conclusions to fit their prejudices and needs. Scientists demand evidence and find very little, but practitioners see improvement in their patients following surgery. With the operation they have settled an annoying issue directly. The mother no longer brings the sniffling, fussing child in to see them, and she, from her point of view, has finally had something tangible done.

The doctor's position has been summarized recently by two otolaryngologists (Fry and Pillsbury, 1987): "But beyond these few stringent protocol criteria, we are mentally paralyzed by the absence of truly prospective, randomized, controlled studies on which to base our decision. We instead begin our careers treating according to the dictates of our original training programs or our interpretations of the massive literature currently available and finally respond to personal judgment."

So it's a matter of personal judgment or the *art* of medicine. And the doctors do make more money doing the operation than by giving pills and reassurance. T&A must still provide otolaryngologists a significant part of their steady income, unless they are heavily into middle-ear ventilation— for which see below.

I don't think money is the important issue for most surgeons, however. More important may be the surgeon's fear of losing his patient and perhaps his referral source. If a patient is referred to him as a possible candidate for a tonsillectomy, he senses the referring doctor's wishes. Though the surgeon insists on making his own decision and his own recommendation, he is biased toward doing the surgery, in most cases, just by the referral.

The parents usually accept the doctor's recommendation of surgery uncritically. In fact, they often bring the child in with the idea of T&A in mind. John Fry, an English practitioner, who was a staunch opponent of the operation, recommending it only forty times in ten years, admitted that parental pressure was the main indication for the operation in six of the forty cases (1957). He could not resist the pressure, he said. Had the children become a sacrifice to their parents' needs?

Is the operation a sacrificial ritual? It was called a prophylactic ritual by the Medical Research Council of Great Britain in 1938 (Fry, 1957). Later, in 1969, R. P. Bolande, an Ohio physician, suggested that T&A and circumcision, where the evidence is even clearer, represent "rites of passage," as described by anthropologists. Many such rites have been surgical, and ritual procedures are often performed on the very young— five years is the most common age for T&A.

If T&A were first proposed now in a time of controlled tests and growing therapeutic caution, it might find little use. The burden of proof would be on those who proposed it. But now the operation isn't so much proposed; it just endures.

As with any medical treatment, you, the customer, have the final say. You would rarely be wrong if you just refused T&A. At least question its use. You might be surprised at how quickly the doctor who recommended it is willing to back down. If you do decide to go ahead, make sure that the surgeon is board certified to do surgery, and that the surgery is performed in an accredited hospital. Following those criteria, the operation may still be unneeded, but at least it will be relatively safe.

CIRCUMCISION

Parents who partake of one ritual operation may indulge in another. Circumcised boys, for example, are seven times more likely to have undergone tonsillectomy than uncircumcised boys (Bolande, 1969). Says Joseph Campbell (1988) in *The Power of Myth*: "In the biblical tradition we have inherited, life is corrupt and every natural impulse is sinful unless it has been circumcised or baptized."

In the instances when circumcision is an avowed ritual (only 2 percent of the cases in one study), it's beyond our consideration here, but its use shortly after birth, with the intention of promoting better adult hygiene, to prevent penile cancer, and to prevent cancer of the uterine cervix decades later in the mates of these males is considered unjustified by most authorities. A committee of the American Academy of Pediatrics reported in 1975, "There were no valid medical indications for circumcision in the neonatal period." The American College of Obstetricians and Gynecologists agreed.

A similar American Academy of Pediatrics committee in 1989 has retreated from this strong condemnation, however, by saying that "newborn circumcision has potential medical benefits and advantages, as well as disadvantages and risks" (Parachini, 1989), the change apparently based on incompletely accepted evidence that circumcised male infants have fewer urinary tract infections. The committee says, in mealy-mouthed justification, that the benefits and risks must be explained fully to parents of newborn boys. Truth is, the benefits are vague.

Medical indications have been proposed on prophylactic or hygienic grounds: Prevent cancer of the penis, cancer of the prostate, venereal disease, and inflammation of the glans (particularly if you live in the desert); prevent cancer of the uterus in sexual mates. Since the AIDS scare one urologist (Fink, 1986) has proposed that presence of a foreskin might predispose to catching AIDS. Critics immediately attacked this undocumented hypothesis, and the most recent American Academy of Pediatrics committee report ignored it.

Army physicians, in a 1986 report, noted a decreased incidence of urinary tract infections in circumcised infants (Wiswell and Roscelli, 1986). But critical rejoinders to this report pointed out that the data were poor, with uncertain endpoint determination and lack of the random, blind design the study needed. In response Wiswell, coauthor of the original work, said that a "long-term prospective evaluation" is needed. So it goes. When you get pushed into a corner, call for an expensive, long-term, multicenter study. Many of these called-for studies are never launched.

Because evidence for these medical indications has been weak or nonexistent, and because simple cleanliness seems a more rational solution to any of them than circumcision, most clinicians who have spoken up conclude that there are no absolute medical indications for routine circumcision in the newborn. If phimosis (inability to retract the foreskin) does appear, it should be taken care of later.

Intending to look into this tenuous evidence to support a formerly discredited operation, the American Urological Association has appointed a Circumcision Study Group, and the California Medical Association's policy-making body has gone further by voting to endorse a resolution calling circumcision "an effective public health measure" (Parachini, 1988). Is voting the way to settle matters that might be resolved by scientific inquiry? There is still no good medical evidence for routine circumcision in newborn infants.

P. J. Zimmer, writing about modern ritualistic surgery (1977), estimates that one seventh of males worldwide are circumcised, but a far greater proportion than that have had the operation in this country—80 to 90 percent before the 1970s. Despite extensive parent-education efforts advising against the operation, most male newborns continue to be circumcised in the United States—over 58 percent by one estimate.

As one of the oldest known surgical procedures and the only elective operation performed routinely without anesthesia, circumcision often falls into the hands of unskilled operators—interns, medical students (Stang et al., 1988). Yet the operation employs special and rather complex clamps that require experience for deft use. If circumcisions are to be carried out, say some obstetricians and urologists, operators should be trained, and the operation should be done as humanely as possible with local anesthesia. The infant fusses less, cries less (in his helpless state his only way of objecting), and obviously has less pain.

Complications are rare, but as with any surgery, existent. Fifteen percent bleed. Infection, septicemia, hemorrhage, mutilation of the penis, and stenosis (a narrowing or constriction) of the penile opening are other reported complications. Rarely the entire skin of the penis or the penis itself has been lost. All deaths due to circumcision—no deaths reported in recent years—have been traced to infection, a preventable complication (Grossman and Posner, 1981).

Though its fee per operation is modest, a few hundred million dollars a year could be saved by stopping circumcision. Taking this matter into their own hands, some third-party payers are now refusing to pay for circumcision (Schoen, 1987). Could it be that the American Academy of Pediatrics committee, as representatives of an underpaid specialty, have, by means of their recent tentative approval, hope of reinstating third-party payments?

Some who study circumcision's use say that the decision whether or not to circumcise a baby is almost entirely a cultural—as opposed to a medical—issue. No one predicts that this operation will disappear.

Middle Ear Ventilation

"Fluid in the ear, glue ear, and conductive hearing loss have replaced the 'infected, large, or hypertrophied tonsils' and 'enlarged adenoids' as a major concern of primary physicians caring for children and the special domain of ear, nose, and throat physicians," says Gunnar B. Stickler of the department of Pediatrics, Mayo Clinic (1984). Small children who formerly submitted to a T&A (and in some places still do) now have their middle ears "ventilated" with small plastic tubes placed in the ear drum—an operation introduced in 1954 that only achieved its peak after T&A began to fade.

Is it needed? In most cases probably not, but kids with stuffy noses and earaches are a big business for children's doctors, who, if they are surgeons, have been in retreat since the start of the antibiotic era. They keep coming up with inventive, new, mechanically sensible operations that don't, however, ever seem to acquire sufficient rational, supporting, clinical evidence. Early in the antibiotic era, they lost mastoidectomy, but T&A remained a stable preoccupation until wave after wave of criticism finally slowed their assault. Now, while they have one third or fewer T&As than during peak years, middle-ear ventilation has come to their rescue. Lumped together the two surgeries—T&A and middle-ear ventilation—probably furnish them more business than they have ever had.

A middle-ear ventilation intends to treat persistent otitis media (accumulation of fluid in the middle ear). A cold or sore throat often blocks the Eustachian tube (a tube which leads from the middle ear to the back of the nasal cavity), and this blockage prevents the middle ear from draining properly. Germs may thrive in the stagnant middle-ear space. Middle-ear pressure increases, producing earache, and the resulting illness, otitis media, may affect hearing when the accumulated fluid prevents the eardrum from vibrating normally. The disability abates, however, as over months or years the effusion clears naturally.

Half of all American children by their first birthday, and nine of ten by their sixth, suffer at least one attack of otitis media. It accounts for about 26 million visits to doctors each year and an annual American medical and surgical cost of at least $1 billion (Gates et al., 1987).

MEDICAL TREATMENT

Antibiotics given for at least ten days are the first line of treatment for ear infections (Mandel et al., 1987). Usually the infection clears, but fluid sometimes remains trapped in the middle ear, target then for a new cold or sore throat that reactivates the infection. Fluid remaining may impair hearing—possibly, some say, to frustrate learning.

INDICATIONS FOR SURGERY

Some investigators have identified a correlation between persistent middle-ear disease with hearing impairment and delays in speech development, language skill, and cognitive skills (Olsen, 1986). Other authorities believe, however, that children can overcome or compensate satisfactorily for mild, temporary hearing losses. Dr. J. L. Paradise of Pittsburgh, whose studies on the effectiveness of T&A I have mentioned, finds evidence extremely weak that persistent fluid in the ears can cause lasting learning handicaps (Brody, 1986).

In any case, as Dr. Olsen, an advocate of tympanostomy, says, "The known and proposed mechanisms that link Eustachian tube dysfunction with serious otitis media are complex and not permanently corrected with a tube or grommet" (1986). All disputants seem to agree that growing up puts an end to the problem of middle-ear infections and persistent fluid.

Olsen says, further, that he and his associates use it in three groups of patients: (1) those with significant hearing loss from middle ear fluid, who fail to respond to antibiotics after a prolonged period of time, (2) those with uncontrolled infections of the middle ear, (3) those who suffer complications of acute otitis media. They make no reference to learning defects as an indication.

J. L. Paradise says, if all infection has been eradicated and the fluid persists, wait three months to see if it clears up on its own—longer if improvement is apparent. A longer wait is also justified if the child's hearing is not impaired and if summer is coming, since warm weather generally brings at least a temporary halt to ear infections. If at the end of three months the child still has fluid in the ear but has no infection and is otherwise healthy, he recommends a simple myringotomy to drain the fluid. If the fluid remains after six months with no signs of improvement, then a tube may be the best remedy.

THE OPERATION

Chronic middle-ear effusion has been treated by myringotomy, adenoidectomy, placement of tympanostomy tubes (middle-ear ventilation), and even tonsillectomy. The surgeon hopes to drain the fluid in the middle ear and prevent its reaccumulation. Myringotomy alone—a little slit in the eardrum—allows the fluid to drain, but the slit soon closes, and fluid recurs in 40 to 50 percent of the cases.

For a middle-ear ventilation, the surgeon inserts a tiny tube into an eardrum slit, usually in an ambulatory setting without admission to the hospital. It permits continuous drainage for as long as the tube remains in place—a few days to a few years, six to seven months on the average, some remaining as long as seven years. They are allowed to drop out by themselves. The tubes are usually less than 3/16 inch long, with a hole less than 1/16 inch in diameter. This open window into the middle ear compensates for the blocked Eustachian tube that has caused the fluid accumulation.

Should adenoidectomy be added? George Gates of San Antonio believes so (1987). He and his associates studied four groups: myringotomy, tympanostomy tubes alone, adenoidectomy alone, and adenoidectomy with tympanostomy tubes. As measured by hearing acuity and the number of surgical retreatments needed, adenoidectomy with tympanostomy was best. Their indications for these operations were rather stringent and might almost have met Dr. Paradise's indications—wait at least three months—but they used no nonsurgical controls. "Surgical therapy does not cure patients with chronic otitis media with effusion," says Gates, "only time, growth, and development can—but it does substantially reduce morbidity when medical therapy has failed." Theirs was a two-year study which at its end didn't finally favor one operation over another: Proportion of children, or ears, remaining free of recurrence was similar in the various groups.

COMPLICATIONS

In addition to the usual complications of general anesthesia, the child may sustain an infected ear, permanent eardrum perforation, a permanently scarred eardrum, or an accumulation of cholesterol debris in the middle ear (cholesteatoma) (Parella, 1980). Ear infection recurs in 20 to 40 percent of cases after the ear tubes fall out. Some abnormalities, with uncertain long-term significance, have been found after surgery in 32 to 67 percent of cases.

Children may be advised to keep their ears out of water as long as the tubes are in place, but one study of children allowed to go swimming after surgery without using earplugs found no increased incidence of middle-ear infection (Eckberg et al., 1987).

EVALUATION

Dr. Paradise, whom I have quoted before, says, "Many, too many, children are getting tubes. It's like tonsillectomies used to be in the

1940s—every child who walks gets one. For every one child who needs and gets tubes, about twenty others get them who don't need them."

As with many operations we examine in this book, middle-ear ventilation was introduced on hypothesis principally. It makes sense mechanically, as do many new operations. They are introduced and often widely used without being adequately tested beforehand (in the way the Federal Drug Administration requires new pills to be tested). Radical mastectomy, coronary bypass, tonsillectomy are other examples. Controlled studies, if they are undertaken later, always drastically reduce the indications for the procedure.

Olsen (1986), who, as I have noted, supports the operation, is in no mood to wait. "We welcome controlled randomized studies," he says, "yet, until they are satisfactorily performed, we believe that a moratorium on tubes is inappropriate."

Says G. B. Stickler (1984), whose quotation introduced this section: "Confronted with three carefully controlled studies showing no demonstrable benefit from the placement of myringotomy tubes in children with secretory otitis—and indeed showing some complications, such as scarring and permanent perforation—it might be wise to accept the statement presented by the editor of *Clinical Otolaryngology*," who wrote, "Adenoidectomy has been shown not to influence the course of otitis media. An equally valid conclusion is that secretory otitis media is a self-limiting disease, which is not affected by any of the current methods of treatment." In most patients the condition resolves with a tincture of time. Stickler concludes, "Let us declare a moratorium on tube placements until solid data supporting the procedure have been reported."

This, of course, is not likely to happen. The operation may well be offered for your child. You'll have to decide.

18

Experimental Operations

Has your doctor recommended an "experimental" operation? What does he mean? Why not have a for-real operation instead? Doesn't someone know? Don't experiment on me.

Medicine's official voices consider new operations, which are often examples of the halfway technology I mentioned in Chapter 1, to be "experimental" until some Consensus Development Committee appointed by the National Institutes of Health (and usually loaded with members who have vested interests in accepting the operation) proclaims them to be "therapeutic." The NIH doesn't want regulations, you see; it just wants a "clarifying of the state of the art," a laying-out by authorities of the base upon which others may act (Perry, 1978). Once the operation has been labeled therapeutic, insurance companies, Medicare, and other third-party payers may be expected to start paying the bills for it, and you might be inclined to submit—but cautiously, I hope.

Operations for obesity, as an example, have been experimental for years—and still are. Artificial heart installations, though they had titillated the media enormously, can hardly be justified as even adequate for human experimentation—they are surely not "therapeutic." Some kinds of transplantation operations (kidney, heart) have in some environments moved from the experimental into the therapeutic range. Any operation, however, having by means of committee decision become "therapeutic," is not necessarily adequately validated scientifically. So do be wary.

Keep in mind, too, that you may encounter different meanings of the word "experiment." The laboratory study and technical invention of an operation and then, if promising, its clinical testing are essential steps, correctly designated as *experiment* or as *experimental testing*. Properly carried out, these steps may come up with evidence that justifies further testing or acceptance of a new operation. Or results of these preliminary steps may, at any stage, force the operation's advocates to discard what at first sounded like a good idea. This kind of experimental testing is essential to sound medical practice.

In another meaning, a doctor who recommends an operation that he isn't very sure about may describe the operation as an "experiment," as a good (but no doubt ill-defined) chance that it might help—"fifty-fifty," say, or something like that. In this case, think of it as just *his* experiment, his hunch. Say no, go someplace else, or just go home. Unless you are desperate, stay clear of that kind of experiment. Furthermore, as a general rule, avoid any experiments unless they are parts of well-defined, prospective clinical tests, usually carried out simultaneously in many clinical centers. I have mentioned such tests in other chapters and will describe them later in this chapter. If it is such a test, be sure you understand what you are getting into. Listen to the explanation, ask questions. Your informed consent is required, but unless you probe, everything you ought to know doesn't always come through clearly.

Why should we have "experimental" operations in the first place? Henry Beecher, a student of medical research, said in 1970, "The well-being, the health, even the actual or potential life of all human beings, born or unborn, depend upon continuing experimentation in man. Proceed it must; proceed it will. The proper study of mankind is man." This may daunt someone facing the prospect of surgery, but modern surgery, a new and rapidly changing technology, whose innovators come up with fresh schemes all the time, starts with experiment. Some operations, in truth, never get beyond that.

VALIDATION OF AN OPERATION

When a surgeon sets out to devise a new operation, the operation ought to be first of all anatomically and physiologically reasonable. It should make sense according to what we know about the body, how it is built and how it functions. Most physicians have been skeptical of acupuncture because they know of no specific, significant anatomical or physiological connections between a spot on the ear lobe, say, and some distant, malfunctioning organ—it makes no anatomical or physiological sense.

On the other hand, to open up or bypass a narrowed artery supplying blood to a vital organ such as the heart does make anatomical sense. But anatomical sense, though necessary, is frequently not sufficient justification. If the arterial narrowing is just one manifestation of a general disease, surgery will not halt the disease. The bypass itself may soon fail, or suffer invasion by the general disease. It may never carry enough blood to make a difference. In addition to making sense, the operation must work. More study is needed.

EXPERIMENTAL SURGERY

Surgeons with a bright idea head for the dog lab, where an operation is most clearly experimental and the first logical step in following up a bright idea. Beginning with John Hunter, experimental surgery's eighteenth-century founder, surgeons chiefly, and all of us indirectly, have depended on animal-laboratory work for the design, redesign, and first-stage testing of surgical methods. The technical design of surgery and the way it alters function has been worked out in the laboratory with animals who also have benefited from such experiments. Every kind of open heart surgery, the heart-lung machine itself, suturing of blood vessels, removal of the bowel, organ transplantation, nerve repair, and in fact almost every modern surgical operation and technology had to survive development and testing in the experimental laboratory. Better to start with animals than with you or me: This, an enduring principle of the profession, is not apt to be overturned by the Animal Rights Movement. In the laboratory, where many surgeons, including me, learned the craft, ways to insure survival and recovery are investigated and altered function analyzed. Surgeons practice. I'd rather have a surgeon make his first, inevitable, technical blunders on a dog than on a person. In the lab an operation can be refined, not to the point where you can be sure it will be useful in man, but to the point where surgeons can perform it in man with some confidence. It must finally be tested on man.

CONVENTIONAL CLINICAL TESTING

The traditional method of testing a new operation in man seemed reasonable. Surgeons who had invented, or were inclined to try, the new method would use it on willing patients, then compare their results with the results of former operations or competing treatments. If their results were better, they would write papers, give speeches, proselytize. Simple enough, but the process typically grew more complicated. Other surgeons would disagree and respond with their own reports, based on the new operation, on older operations, or on different new operations or treatments. Disagreements might lead to "schools of thought" founded on weak scientific evidence. Arguments might endure unsettled for years. In time, some or all of these competing operations, even the temporarily triumphant, might be dropped, forgotten by all except possibly those still living with their ill effects. (See abandoned operations in Chapter 2.)

Or this conventional clinical testing method would amass a great amount of uncontrolled evidence from many sources over a long time, then perhaps achieve a consensus that, with more careful testing, would finally have to be abandoned—radical mastectomy for breast cancer is a good example. In that case a consensus that lasted for eighty years had finally to be forsaken. Thoughtful investigators began to realize that they should, and finally could, employ a more rigorous scientific analysis of clinical data.

The conventional method's experimental design contrasted sadly with the elegant, biostatistical experimental design which had been applied brilliantly early in this century to test such things as agricultural crop yield and basic-biological-science problems. Biostatistical designs came late to clinical medicine because physicians did not understand them, did not believe that they were necessary, or did not, in some cases, feel that a patient should be used as an experimental subject. A patient, after all, is not an insentient plant or a colony of bacteria. Furthermore, there were, and still are, complex problems faced in trying to apply these methods reliably to idiosyncratic, diverse, self-willed (but finally consenting) patients. The struggle is by no means over, but it has gone well enough to create, in the randomized prospective clinical test, a superior yardstick for modern clinical medicine.

IGNORANCE IN MEDICINE—SCIENCE, OR ART?

But do we really need this "prospective clinical testing?" Aren't there simpler ways of deciding what is best? Often there aren't. In a doctor you want more than a scientist, of course; you want a sympathetic, understanding physician who pays attention to all your needs, but you also want a physician who knows what he's doing, someone who has a grasp of pertinent medical science. You don't want to fool around. Prospective clinical testing won't add to our store of sympathetic physicians, but when it works, it may provide your physician with medical science pertinent to your problem—usually for the very first time. It's a fresh wind that has blown away some of the fog of traditional medical practice.

Although the profession has achieved its greatest successes using scientific method, medical ignorance remains widespread and profound (Dykes, 1974). Among its very few true cures are what has been called medicine's high technology—the successful immunizations, the successful anti-infective agents, hormones or vitamins for patients who specifically lack them, and a few curative surgical operations (see Chapter 2).

Fine, we applaud high technology, but if the operation works—I mean if it works for me—why worry? Why bother with all this "science"? I want to get better now; let scientific medicine take care of itself—later. Okay. As you wish, follow your hunch, or someone's hunch—medical independence is our creed.

H. L. Mencken (1927) stated our medical-independence creed in his essay on chiropractic: "I believe that every free-born man has a clear right, when he is ill, to seek any sort of treatment that he yearns for. If his mental processes are of such a character that the theory of chiropractic seems plausible to him, then he should be permitted to try chiropractic." Or anything else, I might add. We allow the sale of cigarettes with no more than a warning label on the package. Why try to control medical treatments?

Doesn't matter very much in most cases. Backache, for example, or any lingering debility that's apt to heal itself in time is doubtless cared for as well, and probably cheaper, by fringe cults as it is by scientific medicine.

When it comes to a surgical operation, however, you may not want to diddle around. All surgery carries some risk, however small, of death or complications. Surgery should have scientific evaluation and open disclosure of the results. A concept naively simple? Why then have we been fooled in the past?

Doctors mean well, don't they? Why are we misguided? One reason: Although most doctors think of themselves as scientists, or at least allied to science, they often prefer anecdote to numerical data. After all, medicine is an "art," and every doctor has his personal experience to go on. But experience, unfortunately, is too often merely the repetition of error. Doctors trust the single case history, the anecdote—their case or someone else's. With that kind of trust, one can jump illogically from the first case to the next case, or perhaps leap upward from one case to a grand generalization.

Leon Eisenberg (1977), a psychiatrist, lists these factors among reasons for the persistence of medical error: venality on the part of physicians, professional incompetence, and lack of commitment to the public weal. But a more important source, he thinks, is the doctor's conviction that what he does is for the patient's welfare. When good evidence is lacking, the best and most dedicated of us do wrong, he says, in the utter conviction of being right.

In addition, both the doctor and the patient may be fooled by the way we humans recover naturally from most illness, mistakenly attributing recovery to the treatment that was going on at the time.

Other barriers between us and the truth are the enthusiasts for any therapy, the zealots trying to convince us. The sheer quantity of biased data they produce from poorly controlled trials may give the illusion of success. Large amounts of poor data tend to preempt any amount of good data.

Plenty of roadblocks, yet there is hope. For as D. P. Thomas said when discussing the matter of experiment versus authority (1969): "There need be no division between clinical and scientific medicine if we are willing to admit our ignorance regarding therapeutic measures, and are prepared to test our hypotheses properly."

PLACEBO EFFECT

It's no easy job to "test hypotheses properly." J. B. Conant pointed this out for science in general in *Science and Common Sense:* "The stumbling way in which even the ablest of scientists in every generation have had to fight through the thickets of erroneous observation, misleading generalizations and unconscious prejudice is rarely appreciated by those who obtain their scientific knowledge from textbooks."

If we narrow this down to clinical science, the testing which Thomas calls for becomes difficult for several specific reasons. One reason, particularly onerous in surgery where it has seldom been carefully identified or fully acknowledged, is the placebo effect.

The term "placebo" has been used since the early nineteenth century to specify a medicine given more to please than to benefit the patient (Beecher, 1955). Its effect has been described as "the effect of any therapeutic procedure or component thereof which objectively does not have any specific activity for the condition being treated." Dr. Albert

Schweitzer, when asked how he could account for the fact that anyone could possibly expect to become well after having been treated by a witch doctor, said, "The witch doctor succeeds for the same reason all the rest of us succeed. Each patient carries his own doctor inside him" (Cousins, 1977). That too may be called a placebo effect.

These definitions refer to a psychological reaction rather than a clear pharmacological effect. If you wanted to take something that would cure your heartburn, for example, you might try Tums because you thought the chemicals in the pill would neutralize the stomach acid you assumed was causing your indigestion—a physiological effect. However, if someone gave you a pill that looked okay but contained nothing but sugar, and your heartburn disappeared promptly, that would be a placebo effect. Thus, we speak of placebos as sugar pills. But doctors don't give sugar pills nowadays. In fact there is no pill in the *Physician's Desk Reference* listed as a placebo. Instead, doctors give drugs like Valium, which have a physiological action, but in addition, produce a placebo effect, important but uncertain in magnitude. Any "pill, potion, or procedure" may have a placebo effect as an adjunct to its intended pharmacological or mechanical effect.

How does it work? Modern neurophysiology searches for a physical-chemical source of any psychological event. The brain, is, after all, a meat machine. In this vein we do now have a tentative, partial explanation. The narcotic antagonist, naloxone, which can block the effect of drugs like morphine, can also block the pain-alleviating effects of placebo pills in about a third of patients—a finding suggesting that placebos may cause the release of the body's own internal painkillers, the morphinelike endorphins. Precisely how they might do this is not clear.

Placebos relieve wound pain, the pain of angina (heart trouble), headache, seasickness, cough, mood changes, and anxiety. About one-third of patients have a high degree of relief of subjective complaints from placebos; on the other hand, they don't seem to work in about one-third (Beecher, 1955). They are an inseparable part of medical treatment, with, by the way, their own side effects.

Surgery, too, has a strong placebo effect. In the experiment for coronary artery surgery summarized in the next paragraph, most of the patients in the placebo group had relief. However, without far more experimental evidence than we have, we can't tell just how strong the placebo effect of surgery will be or for whom it will work best. Ideally, new operations should be subjected to clinical tests, using randomly selected test and control groups and a double-blind plan, in the way new medicines are tested before acceptance. This worked in a thirty-year-old experiment that I described in Chapter 3 (Beecher, 1961).

On the basis of flimsy evidence that tying off internal mammary arteries (arteries which run parallel to the breast bone) would divert blood flow to the coronary arteries of the heart, surgeons performed this rather simple operation, under local anesthesia, in patients with angina who then reported striking improvement. But two groups of skeptics, with the informed consent of a few patients, tied the arteries in half of them, selected randomly, did a similar operation in the other half but without tying off the arteries—a "sham" operation. Most of the patients in both groups reported improvement. The mere act of the operation (no more than a skin incision in the control group) had relieved the pain. After these results were reported, surgeons, who should have been blushing in embarrassment, promptly abandoned the operation. Only on the surgical scene for a couple of years, it would have disappeared even sooner had someone done a controlled study at the beginning.

A decade ago surgeons in Denmark carried out a comparable clinical test on patients with Ménière's disease—one-sided ringing in the ear, deafness, and dizziness associated with fluid accumulation in part of the inner ear. Patients who had a placebo operation—sham operation—responded as favorably as those who had the test operation. There is, say the experts, "a large psychological element" in Ménière's disease. So what's new? This "large psychological element" often runs rampant on the medical—and surgical—stage.

When commenting on the placebo effect of surgery twenty-eight years ago, Henry Beecher (1961), the anesthesiologist I have referred to before, said, "Difficult as it is to carry out controlled study of extensive surgical procedures, the truth often cannot be arrived at acceptably without it, that is, without undue cost in money, time, suffering, and life itself." He went on to say, "One may question the moral or ethical right to continue with casual or unplanned new surgical procedures—procedures which may encompass no more than a placebo effect—when these procedures are costly of time and money, and dangerous to health or life."

Beecher made sense, but surgeons have carried out few controlled surgical studies such as the internal-mammary-artery-angina study. The important breast cancer studies I described in Chapter 9 were indeed controlled studies, but they did not require a sham operation because cancer recurrence or death were the end points. However, if relief of symptoms or improved "quality of life" (results in which the placebo effect is sure to count) become the surgical end point, a controlled test with a sham operation might be the only way to clear the air.

In order to test the angina operation, surgeons used a low-risk, minor sham operation. A major operation evaluated in this same way would require a major operation as its matching sham operation, perhaps something as perilous as an abdominal exploration or a chest operation. Thus, we see that at some point science would carry us too far. Any major operation, sham or not, carries a major risk. Even if patients would volunteer for such an experiment, few surgeons would think of carrying it out, for it would violate their traditional ethic: Do not risk harm when there is no expectation of help.

Many surgical operations have not required a controlled clinical test for validation. Some, even at inception, have hardly been what we would now designate as an experimental operation. Faced with the problem of correcting a potentially fatal congenital defect, for example, the surgeon's challenge was that of devising a way of making the repair effectively and safely. It didn't take a controlled test to prove that closing an abnormal opening between chambers of the heart was a good operation any more than it took a controlled test to prove that streptomycin was a good treatment for tuberculosis meningitis. Without repair the congenital defect was ultimately fatal; without streptomycin the meningitis was quickly fatal. One critical success may be enough.

Practically, acceptance without controlled testing applies when physical correction of a diseased state is the primary problem. If a surgeon can lastingly repair a hernia, he has probably done a good operation. Removing a piece of obstructing cartilage from a knee joint may need no controlled clinical test—though you might want to compare one technique with another by some means. Broken bones must be set, wounds closed; we find many examples.

CLINICAL TRIALS—PROSPECTIVE RANDOMIZED CLINICAL TESTS

The first randomized clinical test, reported in 1948 as a test of streptomycin for the treatment of pulmonary tuberculosis (Freiman et al., 1978), proved convincingly that streptomycin could cure TB. Since then, like the first one, most prospective clinical trials have been with drugs, not surgical operations.

Here, briefly, is the protocol of a modern controlled clinical test:

Patients are divided by random choice into a test group and a control group, and the first group is given the drug being tested and the second a placebo, usually sugar pills or injections of saline. Neither the patient nor the examining doctor knows who is getting what, the drug or the placebo. Thus the term "double blind." At the end, those who evaluate the test try to provide an unbiased assessment. To be accepted, the drug must be significantly better than the placebo and better than older treatments, if they are part of the test.

As a consequence of such tests, drugs once thought to be effective have been abandoned; others have found a firm place in the therapeutic armamentarium. We never achieve certainty, though probability does increase.

ETHICS OF THE CLINICAL TRIAL

Basic to a physician's ethic is his intention never to harm his patient unless there is the possibility of benefit, but experimentation may violate that ethic. A subject may be harmed with no expectation of personal benefit. Should we therefore avoid the experiment? Impossible! Essential to medicine's great theme of progress, experimentation must continue. Thus we have the roots of an ethical dilemma.

Not too long ago medical educators were quietly content to transmit medical ethics by choosing who they thought were morally reliable students, pointing out the Hippocratic Oath to them (first of all do no harm), and then teaching by example. But these educators now face new and revived ethical challenges, unprepared. They have responded by adding a new breed called "medical ethicists" to the faculty, but critical issues trouble this new breed and anyone else who regards the medical scene. A decade or so ago several examples of the scandalous and unnecessary use of uninformed patients as experimental subjects came to light. Respected cancer investigators were caught injecting live cancer cells to uninformed geriatric patients. A group of uninformed black subjects with syphilis went untreated for decades so that progress of their disease could be observed (Barber, 1976).

More recently, in the face of massive technological, life-sustaining achievement, the patient's "right to die" has reached a critical ethical-decision level. The question of when a deformed infant should be sustained, perhaps with a transplant, is fanned by news reporting. The argument of "right to life" or "prochoice" reaches the highest political levels. Should fetal remains serve as transplant farms? There is more: Now philosophers predict that we cannot indefinitely offer high-level, enormously expensive therapy to the very old. Every year, if not every season, brings forth new ethical dilemmas.

Among these are the ethical dilemmas introduced by the prospective clinical test. The first users of a new treatment or a new operation are always experimenters. Both the old, *ad hoc* method of just trying something new to see if it worked and the modern prospective clinical trial are experiments. But society's need for experiment may conflict with the patient's need. In his role as doctor to a patient, a physician's ethical commitment is exclusively to his patient. As a scientific investigator collaborating in a clinical test, however, the same doctor has a commitment to the project, a commitment to acquiring scientific knowledge.

As D. L. Sackett wrote in the *New England Journal of Medicine* (1980), "The intervention trial of greatest benefit to patients satisfies three objectives: validity (its results are true), generalizability (its results are widely applicable), and efficiency (the trial is affordable and resources are left over for patient care and for other health research). The first objective, validity, has become a nonnegotiable demand; hence the ascendancy of the randomized trial." If the physician sets out on the randomized trial and then violates its protocol because he feels his patient is not being best served, he may destroy the validity of the whole effort. In that way many patients who in the future may have profited from a valid test may suffer from its failure.

The current resolution of this dilemma sets informed consent as its objective. If the patient fully understands what is going on and then accepts his role as an experimental subject, the responsibility becomes his, say the experts. The experiment may then proceed with proper scientific rigor and statistical precision, though the individual subject is not always best served.

The meaning of informed consent becomes ambiguous, however. Investigators may fear that full disclosure would be an insuperable obstacle to recruiting sufficient volunteers. Some researchers may contend that there is really nothing to choose between the treatments (the purpose of the experiment is to determine if there is), and therefore the patient-subject need not be informed of the random method by which his treatment will be chosen. A patient, however, may want to become part of the experiment only because he hopes thereby to obtain what he believes is a promising new treatment before it becomes generally available. He arrives with a strong bias. If he understands that once he becomes a research subject his treatment will be chosen randomly, he might back out. He doesn't want the placebo or the old treatment, though of course in the end they may turn out to be better than the new treatment.

These dilemmas arise in prospective surgical trials when, as is usually the case, some new operation has been enthusiastically endorsed, publicized, and widely used before a prospective trial. Most people who enter the study have an opinion about the operation. If they want it and fall into the control group, they can, of course, quit the study, return to have the operation later, or have it someplace else. But fortunately for those who don't get the operation, the prospective test seems always to show that the operation is indicated far less frequently than was originally claimed.

THE RECORD OF THE CLINICAL TRIAL

Despite its successes and the way it has changed clinical research, the random, prospective clinical trial has had rough going. It has been criticized because of ethical problems (described above), because of methodological problems, because of expense, and occasionally because of poor design. Sometimes, claim critics, the tests have been discontinued too soon, invalidating results. These tests arouse the resentment of an older generation used to older ways, as well as the objections of New Age believers who harbor a general antipathy to "science."

Control trials alone cannot be expected to define standard therapy, say some critics (Sturdevant, 1977). Judgment must guide a good physician-patient relationship. The "art" of medicine still counts. Trials are expensive, politics may influence their design, and they may require too many people and too much time. A trial to determine whether a cholesterol-lowering diet would reduce heart disease, for example, would take thirty years and have little impact because people have already accepted the idea that it does.

Following the rapid spread of coronary bypass surgery without controlled evaluation, some critics said that constraints on the introduction of new procedures must now finally be accepted (Hiatt, 1977). These constraints have not been applied. An example: Recently, after the report from Mexico of *two* dramatically successful operations for Parkinson's disease (other less successful cases and some deaths not reported), surgeons around the country started to do the operation in what one neurologist has described as an act of "surgical mayhem," (ABC-TV, 1988). Poor results have caused most of these surgeons to abandon the operation, but why did they start?

Surgery has nothing comparable to the Food and Drug Administration to restrain the dissemination of untested operations (Spodick, 1975). The weak mechanisms available for controlling surgeons' behavior are called upon only reluctantly. Furthermore, the challenges of testing new operations are more complex than those of testing pills (Love, 1975; Bonchek, 1979). Consider, for example, that surgeons' abilities vary significantly while pills of a certain kind are uniform. Additionally, surgery keeps changing—the mortality rate, high at first, falls as techniques improve and surgeons gain experience. The product you start testing is altered, unpredictably, during the test. If undertaken too early, a controlled clinical trial might discredit an incompletely refined but still promising new operation.

In a rapidly changing field, the operation under test may be rendered obsolete before the trial is finished. Debate on the merits of coronary bypass surgery remains unsettled while it is being replaced by angioplasty. On the other hand, a randomized study may begin much too late, as was the case for breast-cancer surgery. When should a randomized surgical trial begin?

Investigators trying to answer that question are also trying to define more precisely the role of clinical trails and to create designs that in some cases may lessen the ethical objections. Clinical trials, now an essential research tool, will be improved, but they are not yet fully accepted by the profession.

In a bizarre example of professional objection, a proposal to study radial keratotomy (an operation I have described in Chapter 15) was brought to the courts in two suits (Norman, 1985; Duffey, 1988–89). The defendants were prestigious academic ophthalmologists who had organized a prospective clinical study. Ophthalmologists in practice claimed that they had enough information to judge the procedure safe and effective and charged that by calling the operation "experimental" the academic physicians were trying to shut the private practitioners out of a potentially lucrative area of medicine. They were in violation of antitrust law.

At an average of $1,000 per eye and possibly millions of customers, a lot of lucre was obviously at stake. Also at stake was the issue of how surgical procedures might be assessed before they reach widespread use. Since they are not subject to governmental regulation, the medical profession was expected to exert some kind of control.

They tried. One of the defendants said, "To my knowledge no in-depth scientific peer-reviewed study of the procedure had been conducted, and

hence the safety and efficacy of radial keratotomy was unknown . . .
There was need to verify the claims and document the risks of this largely
untested operation which was being performed on structurally normal
eyes."

Thus began the clinical test, PERK (Prospective Evaluation of Radial
Keratotomy), but by advocating a moratorium on use of the operation its
advocates had effectively shut down radial keratotomy in private oph-
thalmic practice, claimed the plaintiffs. The legal files and expenses grew,
so without admitting guilt, the defendants agreed to pay $250,000 on the
first suit and sign a statement saying that the operation is "effective in
reducing myopia" and in qualified patients should no longer be considered "experimental."

"The basic issue here" pointed out one defendant, "is how should
surgical procedures be brought into the health care delivery system."
Governmental regulation is unacceptable, cooperation among clinicians,
in this case, failed. Would decisions have to be made through a process of
legal confrontation?

No, not yet. The plaintiffs lost the second case but appealed. Then
fortunately, on March 3, 1989, the United States Court of Appeals for the
Seventh Circuit rendered a stinging opinion in favor of the defendants:
"This case should not have gone to the jury; indeed it should not have
gone to trial . . . the remedy is not antitrust litigation but more
speech—the marketplace of ideas." The decision, I am pleased to say,
favored medical science and prospective clinical trials.

The decision only permits the evaluation process, but it does nothing to
protect you against untested "experimental" surgery. It doesn't lessen your
responsibility; you still have to decide whether to accept or decline the
operation. Ophthalmologists may perform, unregulated, as many radial
keratotomies as they are able to line up; some individual surgeons are said
to have done more than 10,000. W. S. Duffey, who described the court
battle (1988–89) summarizes your role: "In this current health care
environment, patients are more and more left to their own resources in
making health care choices."

So much for this new operation, radial keratotomy. New operations are
likely targets for controlled studies. But a number of old "well-established"
operations deserve the scrutiny that a prospective clinical test could bring.
Radical mastectomy, for example, once a well-established operation for
breast cancer, toppled before the evidence of controlled testing. I think
cholecystectomy for gallstones needs controlled study. Hysterectomy

would likely justify several studies. Cesarean section too. Possibly knee surgery for cartilage injury. But for these established treatments randomized controlled studies are too expensive and difficult to organize.

An alternative way of assessing operations that are already part of medical practice has appeared in the studies that J. E. Wennberg (1988) and his associates have made of prostatectomy (Chapter 6). Called patient-outcome research, it brings together published evidence, insurance databases, interviews, and decision analysis in new ways. Already they have upset conventional opinion concerning the relative effectiveness of two operations for benign prostatic hypertrophy.

YOUR RESPONSE

Experimental surgery and, more broadly, science's invasion of clinical medicine are stories with twists and turns that throw authorities into confusion and dispute. These matters can't be simply understood, nor are choices easy. If someone has recommended an experimental operation for you when you are desperate, you may want to go ahead. If it is just a matter of your making a "contribution to science," however, I'd recommend caution. As I think my examples have illustrated, the "science" isn't always that good.

Though I once thought of myself as a surgical innovator, trying to discover and promote new ways, when I had surgery on myself, I was looking for the tried-and-true. When I had cataracts, had my surgeon suggested intraocular lenses—just coming on the scene then—I would probably have said no. Stick with the settled order. The conservative surgeon I chose didn't even make that suggestion. Now, after years of cleaning, inserting, and losing contact lenses, however, I sometimes wonder if that was the way to go.

If you do elect an experimental operation, you should make sure that your case will be part of a serious experimental study. And the issue should be whether or not you yourself need the operation. Be sure you understand its purpose, the risks, benefits, and possible complications. Good luck!

19

Second Opinion

Your insurance company (the payer) is more likely to request—or require—a second opinion than your doctor (the provider). Relatively confident of his recommendation for surgery, your doctor will stand behind it, but insurance companies, troubled by costs, no longer do. When they found that persons with insurance coverage were indulging in much more elective surgery than they had expected, the payers concluded that they were paying for unnecessary surgery. Remedy: Require the concurrence of at least two, maybe more, experts before an elective operation. Now, without a second opinion many payers won't pay, or they pay less.

As medical-expense growth overwhelms them, the payers—Medicare, private insurance companies—in order to save money, have been driven to insist on second opinions. But for you, a second opinion should have the greater value of helping you avoid an unneeded operation.

In 1974 the Health Benefits Research Center at Cornell Medical Center–New York Hospital reported that one in five recommended surgical procedures would not be performed if a mandatory second opinion program were used (McCarthy and Widmer, 1974). With this data a 1976 House Subcommittee on Oversight and Investigation estimated that there were over 2 million unneeded operations a year in this country, causing 11,900 needless deaths (Friedman, 1984).

What's the matter? Are surgeons stupid? Greedy? Yes, I suppose they are at times—human, they have human faults. But they can slip toward unneeded surgery on lesser defects. All it takes is a little surgical bias and a slightly less than exact knowledge in order for them to commit a lot of borderline or unnecessary operations. The wide variation in rates for specific operations from one region to another demonstrates this. In one study of surgical rates for seven common procedures, hysterectomy rates were found to vary sixfold from one place to another; tonsillectomy rates, sixfold; and gallbladder surgery varied ninefold (Stoline and Weiner, 1988). Since the general health was about the same in these various regions, the strikingly different surgery rates demonstrate, though not precisely, different biases, different styles of practice, different amounts of wealth, varying amounts of unnecessary surgery.

Because in the past they have readily reimbursed surgeons for whatever the surgeons chose to do, health insurance plans themselves have been a cause of unnecessary surgery. A client who had to pay from his own resources would probably have shown more caution than one insured. This liberalizing effect of uncritical insurance payment was soon magnified by an oversupply of surgeons, and the rate of inpatient surgical procedures soared by 41 percent from 1971 to 1980 (Schlossberg et al., 1984).

A surgical operation is now performed with greater skill, precision, and basic-science knowledge than ever, but the decision process that recommends an elective operation is far from an exact science. Ben Eiseman, surgeon-author, writing on the *Prognosis of Surgical Disease* (1980), said, "Given the need for precise data concerning the probability of a good or bad outcome following surgical decisions, it is astounding how difficult it is to find such statistics for many common surgical diseases." His contributors to this book complained to him that for their particular field, "You would be amazed how little hard data are available." We have only a little more hard data now than we did a decade ago when that book was written.

Deciding when to recommend an elective operation is an art rather than a science, sometimes merely a guessing game. An elaborate game no doubt, with each patient unique, each patient searching for complex personal objectives that may be reached by the technical achievement or the ritual sacrifice of his operation. If you try to play this game alone, you may soon encounter your limitations. Do consult someone then, someone with a less vested interest than the operating surgeon. Seek a second opinion.

But will the second opinion be more trustworthy than the first? No certainty on that score, rather a dilemma for which a doctor's aphorism may be pertinent: "The problem of calling in a consultant is that you may feel obliged to take his advice."

BUT SOMETHING MUST BE DONE

Economic strain brought about the required second opinion. Something had to be done. It was bad enough to put patients at risk of unnecessary surgery. That recognition itself led to complaints and investigations, but when expenses soared because the medical bite took bigger and bigger wedges of the Gross National Product, bureaucrats and other executives declared a time for action. Insurance companies and the government tried to impose a more stringent diet on the medical glutton. Many schemes appeared (initialed obscurely PSRO, PPS, DRG, PRO), designed to shove the medical industry away from the hog trough. One relatively gentle shove is the second opinion, first advocated and then required. In time, say some medical Cassandras, far more stringent regulations will be imposed—stop funding intensive care of the aged, for example, or for others with diminished social potential. Today we squirm to think of such regulation, and turn instead to tolerable, but probably ineffective, plans for education: Teach the consumer himself to take action.

But what about the profession? Shouldn't it take action, regulate *itself?* Yes, of course, and the profession does regulate itself through licensing boards and board certification. After serious professional infractions, a licensing board will revoke a license to practice—though slowly and infrequently. An incompetent surgeon may be denied hospital operating privileges—though rarely. As a rule the punishment is little more than a tweaked nose or a slapped wrist. The profession and the hospitals, who are usually indistinguishable when working on these matters, haven't done enough. It is difficult to obtain a medical license and board certification, but thereafter control is soft, and continuing medical education is weak.

As in the past, inadequately tested surgery proliferates. The record, cited throughout this book for various operations, illustrates this. The profession's self-control will not adequately protect you from a bad surgical recommendation. More than you'd like to believe, obtaining prudent care is left up to third-party payers, to luck, and to you.

CURRENT STATUS—RESULTS

If it comes from a respected source, a surgeon will note and discuss a second opinion but rarely suggest obtaining it himself. He will, of course, call upon other specialists when he thinks their opinion is needed, but usually not on someone in his own field—at least not formally. I can't remember ever sending a patient off to see one of my professional peers after I had given my—often slowly arrived at—opinion. The stimulus for a second opinion will more likely come from you, your primary doctor, or your insurance company.

The surgeon who makes his recommendation at the end of his decision process tends to consider the process then complete. This doesn't mean that he is deciding without help. If you have seen him more than once, or if you are in the hospital when he makes his recommendation, his decision process may be lengthy. He may discuss your case in detail beforehand with other physicians; your case may have been presented at a hospital conference; he may have searched the medical literature. (None of this is now called a "second opinion.") Finally, prepared to take the responsibility, he makes his own independent decision. A surgeon's aphorism: "The decision for operation cannot be made by plebiscite."

Physician sovereignty, even of this seemingly rational kind, is fading, however. No longer does the physician dictate to you. He is expected to inform you fully, then leave the final decision up to you. The bedrock of medical ethics used to be the physician's best estimate of what is good for your enduring life and health. Today, because of this climate change, it is your informed consent.

Critics object to this new ethic: The physician's acquired knowledge and intent have been put aside too shortly, they say. But I think second opinions for elective surgery do make sense. If there is a difference of opinion on surgery's need and effectiveness, you should know about it and be able to hear the dissenting opinion.

Popular magazines such as *Redbook* and *Better Homes and Gardens* publish articles on second opinions; doctors read learned articles about them in medical journals; third party payers take action. The second-opinion project gains momentum. How is it doing? Have second opinions improved care? Because good care is difficult to assess, we can't be sure; dissenting second opinions may emotionally overload insecure individuals, but they have reduced the incidence of surgery, which was the objective.

For example: In one report of 931 individuals who received a second opinion for urologic surgery, the need was not confirmed on second opinion in 25.7 percent, and most of them (67 percent of them) did not then undergo an operation (Schlossberg et al., 1984). In another study of eighty-eight patients referred for second opinion before CABG, continuation of medical therapy in preference to surgery was recommended in seventy-four (84 percent) (Graboys et al., 1987). Sixty of the seventy-four chose the medical option and did well on it. The authors concluded that a second-opinion policy could reduce the need for surgical intervention in this disease as much as 50 percent.

Second opinion is not always this clearly opposed to surgery, however. In one report of 367 patients who underwent one or two consultations regarding hysterectomy, a whopping 87 percent received second opinions recommending the operation (Easterday et al., 1983). Furthermore, ten of thirteen patients in this study who received two recommendations against any gynecologic surgery still went on to have surgery.

Advocates of second opinions say they are encouraged, nonetheless. As a result not immediately apparent, they speak of a "sentinel effect." It means that a physician will not recommend a marginal operation if he knows the recommendation will be reviewed (Friedman, 1984). Exposed to the criticism of a colleague, he's going to practice more cautiously.

On the down side: "The most striking fact regarding all voluntary second-surgical-opinion programs is that few people choose to use them," says one commentator. If it's up to them, only 2 to 10 percent of patients request second opinions (Krantz, 1986). They go quietly along, lambs to the slaughter.

Because of this voluntary-plan failure, mandatory programs have been picking up steam; those with strong penalties are doing well. In a strong-penalty program, if you should decide to have surgery without a second opinion, the payer will cut or deny your benefits. Less rigid programs may still pay should you choose to have surgery despite a dissenting second opinion. You'll want to check this out with your own plan.

What you really want, of course, is a dependable, accurate, reliable recommendation—for or against surgery. What you get is opinion—first opinion, second opinion. Better than guesswork, folk medicine, or "alternative" medicine in most cases, it would seem, but not ideal. Both opinions could be wrong. Both consultants may be misinformed or unduly biased by their own last case, favorable or unfavorable. They are dealing with inexact knowledge. Any consultant—the first, the second, or any consultant—may have a vested interest in your case, one way or the other, not obvious to either him or to you.

Professional opinion makers are practicing a new kind of medicine on the basis of the new ethics of patient choice. "The belief that patient choice constitutes the basis and primary good for medical ethics is rapidly gaining support among influential physicians," say medical ethicists (Sider and Clements, 1985). You, the patient, are now in charge, or at least you are expected to act as partner in the decision process. Far more fully than in the past, your doctor presents the evidence as he sees it, makes a recommendation, then says it's up to you. The second opinion option as part of this new ethic expects you to use two or more opinions as evidence upon which to base your considered decision. Because the doctors by themselves haven't been doing the best possible job—according to many observers, including many doctors—you are called upon to fill in.

This need has seemed self-evident to many; official American medicine has rapidly accepted it. Others object. R. C. Sider and C. D. Clements, writing in the *Archives of Internal Medicine* (1985), point out that free, rational persons do not always pursue their own good. Patients commonly practice self-destructive, health-risking behavior. These authors say, further, that a patient's preference is not the fundamental criterion for a patient's good. The learning of doctors who spend a long time pursuing the human values of health and well-function should remain paramount. An internist and official of the AMA is reported in the *Wall Street Journal* (*Medicine and Health*, 1987) as stating that the trend toward second opinions "undermines the basic doctor-patient relationship." Doubtless his is a common doctor opinion.

The profession is not settled on the matter, but under the lash of the third-party payers, they can hardly object. Will second opinions help you as well as the third-party payers? is our critical question here. If they can spare you an operation you don't need, I think they will.

HOW CONSULTANTS BEHAVE, AND WHY

Surgeons called upon for a second opinion usually agree with the first opinion. If this means that all surgeons have the same sound, generally agreed upon, knowledge with which to advise you, we have reached an ideal state. This is true for some specific occasions—when you are going blind from cataracts and are otherwise in good health, first and second opinions are bound to agree on surgery. In many instances, though, we haven't reached this ideal state. Opinions are merely opinions, based on fragile information, and the opinion givers might be expected to agree or disagree with one another in many ways.

Surgeons may provide similar opinions because they concur in a systematic error. That is, they may all be wrong at the same time—as they have been many times in the past. Because everyone was doing T&As during their heyday, second opinions would not have halted the mania. Hysterectomy, in vogue today and being pushed by eloquent surgical hucksters, is apt to carry most surgeons along. It's probably okay isn't it? . . . women do want it . . . so, despite the lack of reliable evidence . . . well, what the hell!

Though not always apparent as a characteristic trait of the breed, fellow feeling among surgeons will produce concurring second opinions. Lacking hard data, a second-opinion consultant still has to offer an opinion. Who knows for sure whether the operation is really indicated? Might as well go along and give the first guy the benefit of the doubt. Next time he will be second-guessing me. With no intentional contrivance or intrigue, a "buddy" system takes over, particularly if both consultants work in the same hospital. A "style of practice" develops.

In medical-school hospitals, university hospitals, and in many independent teaching hospitals, the concept of second opinion is, in a sense, part of the tradition. Cases are discussed all the time: on daily rounds, on "grand rounds," before surgery, after surgery. One doctor is finally responsible for the patient's care, but he is supported and criticized by a team of relatively voluble opinion generators. In such a hospital your case receives second opinions without your intervention or request. You may not be fully informed of them or about the dissent they may generate, but they do take place.

Of course this kind of running consultation does not provide the independence of a distant-source second opinion that you may seek by yourself. The teaching-hospital staff—by consensus or by fiat of a chief, by conviction or by experimental design—may have developed a plan of advocating a certain surgical operation, or they may be trying to accumulate experience in something new. Maybe they are off on their own path. They may, for example, resect a colon cancer a certain way or do a special kind of hernia repair. They become experts in their ways. In some cases, especially if your condition is unusual, this kind of expertise may be best for you; but in such a hospital, as in any hospital, the doctors are still dependent on opinion when the evidence is thin—more abundant opinion, perhaps, but still only opinion.

WHY DO PATIENTS BEHAVE AS THEY DO?

Most persons (or is it just most persons who fall into the hands of physicians?) remain docile and accepting. Few choose to seek second opinions unless required to by the payers (Friedman, 1984; Krantz, 1986). They may criticize the medical establishment, bitch about the whole inflated medical enterprise, think of themselves as rational skeptics; but they trust their doctor like idiot children, often with little more justification than that they find him likable, friendly, concerned, and in control. We see individuals travel across the country to a mecca recommended by a mere acquaintance who claims to have had similar complaints now relieved, and then at that mecca accept a risky recommendation unquestioningly. Man's universal quest for guidance may find its quintessential, and sometimes fatal, expression in unquestioning obedience to a physician.

There may, too, in all of us be a taste for sacrifice ungratified until a crisis such as surgery provides the occasion. Or is there in many of us a bit of the strange craving called the Munchausen syndrome (Asher, 1951), a "polysurgical" addiction that drives its victims to seek multiple surgical operations, for which they have actually manufactured indications (hence "Munchausen")? We need explanations. Mary Wright (1986), a psychologist, says that, "Surgery can recycle pain and pleasure experiences, punish for sexual fantasies, treat symbolic fixations, fulfill sadomasochistic drives, serve as a means to try to establish a relationship, be used as a means to avoid something one fears more than the surgery, and, finally, represent a form of symbolic sacrifice." Well! . . . In any case, we do encounter clients who, forgoing a second opinion, readily accept surgery they have learned is often unjustified.

The old system of unquestioning physician trust was reassuring. You may want to stick with it, but be reminded, a few years ago it resulted in a million T&As a year, mostly useless.

WHOM SHOULD YOU ASK
FOR A SECOND OPINION?

Seek someone who knows the territory. For a "surgical disease" such as a hernia, a harelip, or a breast tumor, find a surgeon; for something traditionally managed by nonsurgeons, such as heart disease, peptic ulcer, backache, headache, or ennui, find a nonsurgeon.

Recently a sixty-eight-year-old psychiatrist with Parkinson's disease, to whom a coronary bypass had been recommended, obtained a second opinion from a well-known radiologist. On the basis of this opinion, the psychiatrist decided to forgo surgery. The radiologist was an excellent choice. Many radiologists have a wide knowledge of clinical medicine with little bias in their own practice toward either medical or surgical treatment, so the opinion is a neutral one. If radiologists are willing to take the job, I believe they might more often be used as second-opinion consultants. For the same reason of nonbias, I think that clinical pathologists, who likewise cover the whole field of clinical medicine, would make good second-opinion consultants, though I have no examples to give.

You might ask your doctor or the surgeon he referred you to for the name of a qualified second-opinion consultant, but that route would diminish your independence. Where else? Friends, the local medical association, the local hospital. The hospital will give you the names of qualified specialists on their staff. If you are eligible for Medicaid, you might contact your local welfare office for their list of doctors who accept Medicaid benefits. If you are covered by Medicare, you can find the same information at the local Social Security office.

The Department of Health and Human Services maintains a Second Opinion Hotline: Call 800-638-6833 (800-492-6603 for Maryland residents). Or for a brochure on their Second Opinion program write: Surgery, Department of Health and Human Services, Washington, D.C. 20201. A Second Opinion Hotline is also maintained by National Second Opinion Program, New York Hospital Cornell Medical Center, Health Benefits Research Center. Their telephone numbers are 800-522-0036 (800-631-1220 for New York state residents). For additional information on their program write: Health Benefits Research Center, 235 East 67th Street, Room 201, New York, N.Y. 10021.

Some health insurance plans don't require a second opinion but will pay if you choose to have one. Others reimburse partially; you may have to pay 20 percent of the second opinion fee. Others, in growing numbers, require a second opinion: They pay, and if you fail to obtain a second opinion, they may reimburse you only 50 to 80 percent of surgical costs.

Ask the second-opinion consultant the same questions you asked the first: What are the indications for the operation in my case? What alternatives are there? What might happen if I do nothing? What risks and complications do I face? How much improvement can I get? Tell me the late aftereffects. Level with the guy. Watch for him to blink. Remember, it's mostly opinion; so don't expect the facts you'd really like to have. This is an inexact science.

BOOKS AND LIBRARIES AS CONSULTANTS

You can obtain a second opinion from books—this book is an example— or from health magazines. Eugene McCarthy, whose 1974 article started the second-opinion ball rolling, has written a guidebook on second opinions (1987). In addition, don't be afraid to seek higher authority. Professional textbooks and articles in prestigious medical journals, such as the *Journal of the American Medical Association* and the *New England Journal of Medicine*, are not as hard to understand as you might believe. The summaries that introduce each article are relatively clear and may be all that you need. These articles—referred to throughout this book in parenthetical inserts and listed at the end under "References"—try to present the best available evidence in support of current truth. Much of the criticism I have cited in previous chapters comes from these sources; all of them are open to you.

Medical textbooks are shockingly expensive ($150 for a two-volume production), but along with the journals, they are available to you in medical libraries. The local medical society will probably maintain a library as will the larger hospitals. Medical schools have extensive libraries, and some universities, though they lack medical schools, still carry many medical books and journals in their libraries.

You may just want to look up your particular problem in a surgery textbook, but if you prefer to probe more deeply—let's say find out what has been written since the textbook was published—the *Index Medicus* is the key to medical journals. It comes out each year in multiple volumes and covers current medical literature according to subject or author. In order to use this, you may need a little help from the medical librarian, who, by the way, may also have access to all of this information with a computer terminal that will give any literature search a modern, well-documented, and more expensive air. Most medical librarians are by nature helpful, and many, no doubt due to their intelligent and long-enduring observation of the profession, view it skeptically. Since yours is a skeptical mission, the librarian may go out of her way for you. In any case, she will let you use the books.

ALTERNATIVES TO A SECOND OPINION

Simple trust in your primary doctor and primary surgeon is the obvious alternative to a second opinion. Do what you have been told—the course taken by most patients. In the best of possible (scientific) worlds, your doctor would surely know best, but it doesn't always work out that way for two main reasons: First, the best medical knowledge is incomplete; no doctor knows. Second, individual doctors may base their recommendations on prejudices, misinformation, and old biases—on personal experience and anecdote rather than on sound evidence. Your search for a second opinion is a response to this uncertainty—hardly an ideal response, but more sensible than blind trust in just one opinion.

Doctors often seem to value their personal experience more than the accumulated experience of the profession. But when a doctor's behavior does show up as stubbornly in opposition to available data, we must remember, to his credit, that his opposition to authoritative opinion finds justification in the past mistakes of authorities. Their record is tainted.

Nevertheless, expert opinion is generally the best opinion we have, and reason obliges us to accept its sensible use. This line of thought brings us to a second-opinion alternative called decision analysis—a mathematical technique that produces a recommendation based on objective information from the medical literature. Not necessarily correct, of course, but presumably the best we can do in light of current knowledge. In one comparison study the investigators concluded that decision analysis was preferable to second opinions in verifying surgical decisions (Clarke, 1985), but the technique doesn't seem to have caught the interest of many practitioners yet. It's a little far out in the direction of probability, algorithms, and artificial intelligence.

IF YOU ACCEPT, PLEASE COOPERATE

If your second opinion confirms your first recommendation, and you decide to have surgery, try to lie a little low on any further running criticism. Cooperate. An adversarial doctor-patient relationship breeds harm. Be alert, yes, but don't ask for more vitamins in the IV or new antibiotics. Let the doctors change the dressings and prescribe the enemas by themselves. Let the nurses schedule the medications and the meals.

I remember an irate surgical resident who finally tossed the order book on a patient's bed. (The patient, by the way, was a surgeon—they have bad reputations as patients.) "Here!" cried the resident, "you write the orders, doc." The surgeon-patient, startled, fell back on his pillow, mum. A day's time partially healed the rift, and despite the blowup, the resident continued to write the orders. But following the incident, they gave the surgeon-patient less attention, left him more to chance—in whose care he did recover satisfactorily.

20

Choosing a Surgeon

Said John Hale (1529–68), the ideal attributes of a surgeon are: "Heart of a lion, eye of a hawk, and hand of a woman." This lyrical notion may not help you choose one, or perhaps at this point you have already made the choice or had it made for you. A health maintenance organization, for example, limits your choice, and if you are a group-practice client, you'll find that they have their surgeon waiting.

Still, though limited by these arrangements, you may want to learn something about the professional competence and personal nature of the person who proposes to invade your body. In this chapter I'll describe the training and certification of a surgeon, the ways in which he acquires experience and professional stature, something about a surgeon's nature and personality, the impact of his environment, his type of practice, and the methods you might employ to select a surgeon, for you do have a choice.

If it's elective surgery, the choice of the surgeon can be yours. You can travel to another city; you can change doctors; you can change medical-care systems.

PROBLEMS

But opportunity brings with it problems. Among surgeons, competence varies: some excellent, others mediocre, some bad. Even the best among them may be competent in only a narrow field—a field from which they sometimes wander. If they believe that they need more surgery, they find little in their licensing, their specialty certification, or in hospital control, that restricts them to the area of their greatest competence. They might stray a little, to your disadvantage.

In cities (where most of them practice) surgeons are a growing surplus. Then, because you may have several to choose from, you may consider this helpful, but the surplus also creates a dangerous need of the surgeon to find surgical cases—to operate. No specific authoritative body in the profession or in the government has been charged with providing surgical manpower guidelines. Hence, with no restrictions, their number has increased by 25 percent since 1979 (Rutkow, 1986). There has been no comparable increase in the number of operations done, so we have fewer operations per surgeon, and thus less-experienced surgeons. The surplus of eager, even needy, surgeons continues to grow.

Quality control of surgeons, of all doctors for that matter, is poor—in some environments almost nonexistent. Though relicensing is required, doctors are effectively licensed for life. If on a local level or on a specialty level conscientious doctors try to control quality by peer review, they may run into a legal mess. When medical staffs or hospital governing boards have sought to restrict or revoke the rights of practicing physicians, they have incurred antitrust lawsuits. One of these suits has been fought in Oregon for ten years (Curran, 1987), and another (described in Chapter 18) has, according to the journal *Science* (Norman, 1985), "split the ophthalmology community." Some states have passed laws designed to make peer review legally less dangerous for the reviewers, and federal legislation promises to provide some immunity, but with complex issues to impede action, effective peer review seems a way off.

Their practice now more crowded, competitive, and nerve–racking than ever, surgeons are soon to suffer a loss of income. Following a Harvard Relative Value Study, which favored "cognitive" physicians rather than "invasive" physicians (Booth, 1988), a Physician Payment Review Commission has proposed a basic revision in the way doctors are paid by Medicare. Fees for internists would rise as much as 26 percent to 35 percent, and surgical fees would fall, particularly for twelve procedures previously identified as overpriced: coronary bypass, hip replacement, cataract extraction, prostatectomy, and others. If you have a recommendation for surgery, you clearly face problems. Now you can see that surgeons, too, face many problems.

The surgeon must retain his poise, retain his compassion, and refine his competence. I believe that competence, difficult though it is to estimate, is the first thing to look for in a surgeon. It's built on an individual's natural aptitude, and evolved through training and experience. Medical schools enroll students with natural study aptitudes and good memories, train them to a certain level, and provide them with a bit of experience. Training continues during the residency, and, in the best of circumstances, goes on and on throughout an entire career.

TRAINING

As with any complex maturing process, surgical training is difficult to appraise, but there are certain indicators. The framed diplomas and certificates that some doctors mount on their office walls might inform you partially, but by the time you first see these displays, you're already engaged face-to-face with the actual doctor. The framed paper blurs. Luckily, you can acquire the pertinent information more accurately by asking the doctor himself, by asking his secretary, or by looking him up in the directories I'll list.

MEDICAL SCHOOL

We know that doctors take a long course, as do priests, dentists, lawyers, and aspirants for a vast number of Ph.D. degrees. These courses may all be excessively long, but they do provide employment for professors and many other workers in a higher-education industry, and in the case of a doctor the long course gives candidates time to mature a little. When discussing ways by which medical education might be shortened, an acquaintance of mine defended the long course by saying, "I don't want my wife attended in labor by a doctor who isn't old enough to have had a wet dream."

By the time they have finished the long course, doctors are well beyond the first experience of a wet dream, sometimes clearly past their carnal peak, and old enough, in many cases, to move with middle-aged deliberation—and think in fixed and routine ways.

The course is intended, first, to educate them generally, next, to train them in the sciences broadly, then in sciences basic to medical practice. Finally, near the end they are trained in the clinical, or applied, branches of medicine. About eight years after finishing high school, they receive the M.D. degree. Nowadays most MDs take another three to five years of apprentice-type residency training to become "board certified," as "diplomates" in one of the twenty-three specialties (ten of which are surgical) that approve such training and give certifying exams. Just before or during the residency, they also take exams, given by the individual states or by the National Boards, that license them to practice medicine generally as a "physician and surgeon." A process controlled by the doctors themselves, it is in many respects a model system for training professionals, but it isn't perfect. The training isn't uniform, and no one effectively follows up on the product.

Because they have more qualified applicants than openings, the 127 medical schools in the United States are choosy. They know enough about medical education now so that, aided by entrance examinations, their admissions committees are able to pick candidates who have an excellent chance of graduating. Picking those who will become "good doctors" is a knottier issue.

Who *is* a "good doctor"? Who is competent? This evaluation is the most important issue in the education of health professionals, says an editorial (Martini, 1988). Both the process (what is evaluated now) and the outcome must be measured, but as the editorial states, "The task is phenomenal." Accrediting bodies are interested in the task and making plans—something for the future, perhaps. Their plans won't help you now.

Some American medical schools, usually the long-established schools and those associated with distinguished universities, have better reputations than others—harder to gain entrance, often more expensive. But it's probably pointless for you to sort through your choice of a surgeon on that basis. All the American schools provide an adequate background for surgical residency training.

When you choose a surgeon, you ought, at least, to find out if he graduated from an American medical school. On average, doctors in this country, trained in American (or Canadian) medical schools, are better trained than Foreign Medical Graduates (FMGs). To this flat rule there are, of course, many exceptions. Distinguished leaders in American medicine are graduates of foreign medical schools; Europe, especially, has many world-famous medical schools; great medical discoveries have been made, and new ones are being made, in those schools. Nonetheless, as a rough guide, other matters being equal, I think you are apt to be better off with an American graduate. A second-rate medical school education, common among FMGs, may have been patched during residency training, but FMGs start with a handicap. Many of them (about half now), by the way, are native Americans who could not gain entrance into American medical schools.

Two decades ago after a "doctor shortage" was perceived and a change in federal law relaxed immigration restrictions, a flood of FMGs entered this country. Previously, Asian physicians had found it almost impossible to try their luck here. Just as well, the guardians of American medicine thought, because FMG education had taken place in schools that were only lackluster copies of European or American schools. Though they had great trouble with the licensing exams that American students found easy, many FMGs were licensed. In 1971 Asia provided 67 percent of entering physicians, while countries such as the United Kingdom, France, and Germany, with which we had traditionally exchanged trainees, provided fewer. FMGs significantly changed the demography of American medicine. In 1973, 47 percent of all newly licensed physicians were FMGs, and by 1977, 20 percent of all active physicians in the United States were FMGs. At the present time, about 16 percent of residents in training are FMGs (Crowley, 1988).

They quickly relieved the perceived doctor shortage. Many worked in emergency rooms, government hospitals, group practices, ambulatory surgery clinics, or clinical labs; they held positions as resident physicians, medical staff doctors for companies, or administrators. By now many of them have found their way into the medical mainstream, and more will. The legal restrictions on FMG acceptance keep changing, and today, once again, as a doctor surplus develops, it has become more difficult for foreign graduates to remain and practice here, though they are welcomed as residency trainees (Boggs, 1987).

RESIDENCY

The surgical residencies most coveted are conducted in the principal training hospitals of a medical school, where medical students as well as residents are trained. (Internships have vanished, by the way.) Some are called "university" hospitals, others are veterans' hospitals, public hospitals (the old charity hospitals), or voluntary hospitals affiliated with the medical school. Perhaps equal in quality is residency training at some of the best-known, long-established clinics, such as the Mayo Clinic, the Lahey Clinic, the Cleveland Clinic, the Ochsner Clinic. The famous public hospitals of our major cities still provide excellent surgical training, because, traditionally, these hospitals grant the resident surgeon important operative opportunity and responsibility.

Residency training leads to "certification." Choose a surgeon who at least has board certification—"board eligible" is not enough. "Eligible" may mean that he has flunked the board exams one or more times. A surgical specialist should be certified by one of the ten surgical boards.* Although not guarantors of high quality, boards are a baseline indicator of adequate training.

Following residency there has been little effective testing of enduring competence. Leon Rosenberg, dean of the Yale University School of Medicine (Horowitz, 1988), says that doctors "have been unwilling to identify and discipline physicians who are incompetent, or impaired, and by doing so have suggested to the public that the guild of medicine comes before the responsibility to the patient." A report from the University of San Diego's Center for Public Interest Law contends that California consumers are offered little protection from incompetent doctors by the state disciplinary system (Ellis, 1989).

Doctors have made efforts, however. During the past couple of decades, medical leaders have popularized "continuing medical education" schemes, and twenty-seven states now require continuing education for reregistration of a license to practice medicine, but these programs usually require only attendance at meetings, not examination. Many of the specialty boards have plans, some in effect, to reexamine their diplomates for recertification. The American Board of Surgery, for example, has provided only time-limited certification since 1975. After ten years, a diplomate must pass examinations for recertification or his listing is changed to indicate an expired certification. This requirement may, of course, not turn out to have a very strong disciplinary action on an established practitioner. A surgeon can get by for life, after a fashion, with what he picked up as a resident.

CAREER

The eminence a surgeon achieves during the years of his practice comes to mean more than his training. If he works in a good hospital, belongs to

*The ten specialty boards in surgery are American Board of Urology, American Board of Thoracic Surgery, American Board of Surgery, American Board of Plastic Surgery, American Board of Otolaryngology, American Board of Orthopaedic Surgery, American Board of Ophthalmology, American Board of Obstetrics and Gynecology, American Board of Neurological Surgery, and American Board of Colon and Rectal Surgery.

professional societies, writes scientific papers, matures with experience, and has peer respect, he may be the surgeon you want.

In some communities a surgeon joins the staffs of all, or at least several, hospitals, but in most communities he doesn't need this. He works more efficiently if he can do all his work in just one good hospital. If he works in a hospital that is affiliated with a medical school and he has been appointed to the clinical faculty, he has received notable professional sanction; in that hospital he may be able to focus his interests and become expert in a few areas. You may need such an expert. Is he doing research on the subject? Has he published articles in the medical literature? You can ask these questions of him, of his secretary, or of the doctor who wants to refer you to him. When I am looking for such an expert in a field of surgery with which I am unfamiliar, I go to the local medical library and search through the *Index Medicus* to see who is publishing articles in the field. (See Chapter 19 for literature search.)

As part of their quest for professional distinction, surgeons join professional societies and attend those societies' meetings. Ask what societies the surgeon belongs to. In some communities, particularly the small ones, a doctor gains first-stage professional approval by joining the local medical society; through it he then automatically becomes a member of the American Medical Association. The AMA is less commonly a measure of professional stature in cities and less so among surgeons. Don't require that your surgeon be a member of the AMA. Actually only about 45 percent of all doctors belong to it. Most surgeons belong to the American College of Surgeons, however, and those who achieve special distinction may belong to smaller societies, such as the American Surgical Association.

Since doctors tend to protect one another against critics, you may have trouble finding out if a doctor has incurred professional disfavor. Lack of clients indicates a kind of professional unpopularity, of course, but that deficiency may be the fate of a highly qualified new surgeon in town, or just the inevitable consequence of too many surgeons about.

MALPRACTICE

At one time loss of a malpractice suit, or even the charge of malpractice, might have discredited a doctor. It might yet be prudent for you to stay away from surgeons who have lost malpractice suits, but in the present legalistic climate, where many busy doctors have suffered unjustified legal assault, to have been the target of such an assault should not discredit a surgeon. I know excellent surgeons who, despite their competence, have lost malpractice suits.

A SURGEON'S ENVIRONMENT

Where he works and how his practice functions influences the way a surgeon makes his decisions. For example, if he works with referring doctors—he can hardly avoid this—he pays close attention to the referring doctor's wishes. The fact that you have been referred to him usually implies to the surgeon that the referring doctor thinks you should have the operation. Unless he is the only surgeon around, he can't oppose the referring doctor's wishes very many times without losing that source of referrals. Once an operation has been considered by your doctor, or perhaps merely suggested by you, a momentum builds toward doing that operation—unrelated to any real objective need for it.

If he practices independently under the traditional fee-for-service system, a surgeon doesn't receive income unless he operates. In its favor, this system provides you with the widest choice of surgeons, but the system can also provide you with the greatest risk of unnecessary surgery. To survive financially—and professionally—any surgeon must operate; the pressure to operate becomes greatest under the fee-for-service system. A stark necessity underlies professional decisions.

Group practice ameliorates this necessity a little, particularly for a beginning surgeon. While a solo surgeon has to depend on an inconstant source of referrals from fee-for-service practitioners, the group assures its surgeons a source of referrals. Popular surgeons who have plenty of referrals usually prefer the solo, fee-for-service style, yet many of the well-known medical groups (Mayo Clinic, Cleveland Clinic, Lahey Clinic, Ochsner Clinic, and others) were started by popular surgeons to whom the efficiency of group practice must have seemed compelling. Though a group surgeon may still incline toward surgery for any borderline case, his own income isn't as immediately dependent on it. However, because the surgical fee goes to the group, which then divides it up as it sees fit, the group as a whole does profit from doing more surgery.

If you prefer more freedom of choice, you can break away from a group. Breaking away from a Health Maintenance Plan (HMP), to which you pay beforehand to have your health maintained, may prove more awkward. There may be no need, but if you do go outside for a surgeon, you'll probably have to pay for that surgeon yourself. Surgeons in a HMP, who do not make more money by doing more surgery, probably have less disposition to recommend surgery than do fee-for-service or group surgeons. Perhaps because of the relatively fixed income these plans offer surgeons, however, the most ambitious and the best-known surgeons have not found them as attractive as either solo or group practice.

Surgeons find jobs in government hospitals attractive when the hospitals are affiliated with medical schools. Veterans' hospitals may engage a prestigious staff. The surgeons are provided with assured income, resident assistants, and time to conduct research. As in an academic medical center, the residents in these hospitals assume significant responsibility, to their benefit and to yours too, I must add, if you are critically ill and need moment-to-moment care.

Surgeons prefer practice in well-equipped, city hospitals, but the surgeon surplus has pushed many well-trained surgeons out into smaller community hospitals. Should you accept a small-town surgeon for your operation? You don't have to; you can travel. Though years ago I did some major surgery in small-town hospitals as an "itinerant surgeon"—a fairly common bad practice at the time—I have no recent experience of the smaller community hospitals. I should think, however, that if you are determined to be hospitalized near home, where friends can easily visit and protect you, you might safely undergo relatively common surgery in the community hospital. For anything unusual, complicated, or tricky, head for the big medical center. Recently, in the small city where I live, surgeons lost a million-dollar malpractice suit as a result of trying, unsuccessfully, to perform exceptionally difficult open-heart surgery in a community hospital. Surgeons practicing in community hospitals have been trained to do bigger operations than regularly come their way. If they do get a big case and decide to plunge ahead, they have to operate with no recent experience and a green team.

City hospitals with training residents have to provide training, and surgical residents train by operating on patients. Though a resident may be assisted, or at least carefully watched, by a senior surgeon while he operates, you may not want to be the patient upon whom that exercise proceeds. If that is the case, you could simply avoid surgeons who practice in training hospitals, provided that you have the choice. Charity (now called public) hospitals used to provide some of the most sought-after surgical training because their patients had no choice of a surgeon; residents did most of the surgery. At the present time, university hospitals, public hospitals, veterans' hospitals, and voluntary hospitals affiliated with medical schools are important training centers because they do provide the resident with the surgery he seeks and needs. He can't learn it by just watching. Surgical residents compete perpetually for a turn to operate.

That you may become part of the training system may not be made clear to you—something you may learn only by actually reading that long operative permission form. If you don't want to be part of the training system, talk it over with your surgeon *before* you enter the hospital. Tell him you want him to perform the operation. Or you might want to save the academic medical center for a complex or rare operation. In academic medical centers, senior surgeons make their reputations by doing as many of those complex and rare operations as they can—successfully and in person.

AGE AND SEX

Old surgeons never die, but you don't have to let them operate on you. Psychomotor and visuospatial abilities, say psychologists, deteriorate more rapidly with aging than verbal abilities (Pickleman and Schueneman, 1987). This being so, your old surgeon may talk a good case for himself, but his technical peak has surely passed. He may be your best choice for a second opinion, but for an operating surgeon select a younger man. Plainly, operative skill resides not just in youth and manual dexterity: problem-solving ability, memory, organizational talent, grace under stress, energy, and a complex set of talents and background that result in good judgment are usually more important. If we assume that he once had them, an older surgeon may lose these qualities more slowly than he loses manual dexterity, but, despite his fame and self-confidence, don't let a deteriorating old man operate on you.

Some surgeons, often those who had the highest operating skill in their prime, withdraw by choice as gracefully as they can. Respect their choice; don't plead with them to operate on you. Others have to be torn away from the table by well-meaning friends; else they will operate until they collapse in the arms of their favorite scrub nurse, incontinent and drooling. The god complex infects surgeons as well as psychiatrists at times. A famous surgeon of the first decades of this century was said to insist on operating though he was almost blind. Touch is important in surgery, and he somehow got by with touch—and doubtless very alert assistants.

At what age should you draw the line? Case-by-case, necessarily, but as a broad rule, retirement age in the midsixties makes sense for a surgeon.

For new surgery or something requiring fine technique, such as microvascular surgery, sixty is too old.

Throughout I have referred to a surgeon as "him." This usage can be defended by the weight of numbers as well as by grammatical convenience. Most surgeons are males. With respect to technical aptitude, clinical competence, ambition, or intelligence there is no reason why males should be preferred, but tradition has favored them. The teachers, mostly males, choose students to fit their own image. I think, further, that physical strength has favored males. Men may be able to remain standing—and still conscious—while pulling lustily on an instrument to hold the wound open (the job of a beginning resident) longer than females can. I have often been grateful for an assistant who had the physical bulk and strength to pull while I mucked around inside. (Maybe I should have been lustily pulling while someone with a woman's delicate, healing hand did the repair.) Users of neuropsychological tests to predict operative performance credit women surgical residents with greater verbal skills than men and with equal motor skills, but found them at some disadvantage where risk taking was rewarded (Pickleman and Schueneman, 1987). These were small-sample studies, however.

You are most likely to have a choice of women surgeons in obstetrics and gynecology, pediatric surgery, or plastic surgery. In obstetrics and gynecology, certainly, a woman's viewpoint and possible personal experience will strengthen her qualifications as a surgeon and as a counselor for you. In other areas there seems to be no reason why a surgeon's sex should weigh in your choice.

PERSONALITY

For the difficult technical act of surgery, you need, first of all, a competent technician. No doubt it's reassuring if you find, in addition, a charming friend, someone whose personality suits yours. Perhaps in the way that older patients prefer older docs over younger docs, who may be thin on experience and inflated with this week's technical news, and in the way that fat persons snuggle up to a fat doctor, you'll find comfort with a surgeon whose prejudices and character traits match yours. I prefer a clinical scientist with high technical skill who has a somewhat skeptical frame of mind. We remain a little aloof, but are compatible at core.

By selecting students interested in literature and the arts as well as in science, medical schools try to produce broadly educated doctors these days, in the belief that worldly understanding promotes patient understanding. But keeping up with the profession occupies the mind, and surgeons tend to become narrow, centering their conversation on the work and their wit on hospital incidents or grisly operating-room fantasies. As with athletes—in a sense surgeons are athletes—they focus their thought on the "sport." If you do uncover the personal qualities of your surgeon, you'll have done so by talking to him or by talking to his patients. Their judgment counts on matters of personality—whether he is sensitive, likable (at least to that patient), attentive, and compassionate.

The discontent that many persons have with modern medicine often focuses on a physician's cool, technical, and unsympathetic attitude toward his patients. Norman Cousins (1978) said patients "don't want their doctors to be impersonal and detached super-scientists but finely tuned human beings capable of exquisite sensitivity and tenderness." A patient's quest for such paragons has been aided by several books, usually written by an internist or a family practitioner, telling a reader how to choose a primary-care physician. You must search for character and personality, say these books. It seems that in the opinion of these writers all doctors possess adequate scientific competence. In surgery they don't. If you are to undergo a life-risking operation—and all operations are to some degree life-risking—I think you will want to place professional competence above personality.

I do not mean to say that competent surgeons lack human qualities. They know love and sorrow. In a professional way of giving time and effort, they are more devoted than any physicians I have ever known. Patients of a surgeon will occasionally come to feel that they don't want to lose him and ask him to become their personal, primary-care physician. Now and then a surgeon will accept that role.

There must be a balance between technical skill and human understanding, what Francis Peabody was referring to when he said (Carson, 1977), "The treatment of a disease may be entirely impersonal, the care of a patient must be completely personal." The competent surgeon may veer toward treatment of a disease. Doubtless you would prefer it that way. Patients' needs may call forth great efforts from their doctors, but sick patients—the kind a surgeon regularly works with—are not lovable. Understandably, they become intensely self-centered, incapable in their time of crisis of returning affection. Doctors learn to accept this, but in doing so, they may withdraw a little from the sick patient—an action that may be necessary for personal survival.

Members of a diverse clan, surgeons mature variously, and that makes them hard to pigeonhole. I think it possible, nonetheless, to identify a couple of traits that characterize most of them. As one trait, a good surgeon wants to perform surgery. He enjoys it; it's a great game.

He also likes to work with material things. In order to strengthen his game, he is into the organic and anatomic rather than the psychological or mystical nature of illness. "Cut well, sew well, get well," he admonishes his acolytes. He dislikes making a diagnosis of "functional" or psychoneurotic illness, and most of his patients agree. They hate being tagged with those soft diagnoses when they know there must be something seriously wrong inside (best removed or rebuilt) to cause their very tangible distress.

A surgeon trusts his own observation when evaluating an operation and may claim, for example, that an operation "works in his hands" despite the lack of controlled, experimental data. Though he may be well schooled in the chemistry, physiology, and pathology of disease, he is not, in most cases, a trained, scientific investigator. Rarely does he understand biostatistical method or experimental design. And he is more apt to remember cases that were referred to him too late than to remember those where surgery might have been avoided. Just as the internist will recommend pills, the physiotherapist massage, and the psychiatrist talk, the surgeon will recommend operations.

THE MECHANICS OF FINDING A SURGEON

Listen cautiously to a former patient's opinion of a surgeon; it's apt to be colored by emotional attachment, a lucky outcome, or a single bad experience. The patient, in the human way we all countenance salesmanship or myth, may have been duped by a good actor, a good talker. I've known doctors very popular with their patients who I thought performed only marginally. Practitioners of "alternative" care, as examples—who often stand highly recommended by their patients— infrequently achieve even marginal care by critical medical standards.

I myself have had patients with whom I had seriously blundered tell me how much they admired my handling of their cases, how grateful they were. When they said this, I may have cringed internally, but I didn't tell them that I had squeaked by on luck and their own strong constitutions. Others, for whom I have unexpectedly exceeded my average competence with what I thought were surprisingly brilliant results, have turned away in the end grumbling, never to see me again. Doctors are frequently surprised by malpractice suits: The suing patient seems to be the wrong patient. Serious medical mistakes may escape laymen's notice, while a good try that fails may uncage legal bloodhounds. I believe that patients are often inept critics. *When listening to their assessment of a doctor, be wary.*

The usual advice in books written by primary-care physicians is to choose a primary-care physician first, then accept the surgeon he recommends, most likely someone near at hand. It may work out beautifully, but you don't have to tolerate this rigamarole even on a local level unless you want to, and of course you may always look afar. If you know that you want an operation—to have a mole removed, say, a hernia repaired, a bleeding stanched, or a nose straightened—you'll save yourself time and trouble by going directly to a competent surgeon. Before operating, he'll make sure you are fit to stand the surgery, and he might spare you the discovery of unrelated, unthreatening abnormalities that the primary-care physician digs up during his "checkups" and "screenings"— often the beginning of much iatrogenic (doctor-caused) trouble. If you have a surgeon you trust, you might also go to him directly for other complaints, for something that may or may not require an operation, but in this instance you could become victim of his strong propensity to "cut it out when in doubt."

Choose a surgeon by reviewing the data I have discussed above: training, board certification, professional societies, hospital staff appointments, publications, and type of practice. These data are available to you by asking, if convenient, the referring physician, the surgeon himself, or his secretary. Medical libraries have directories* that list this information—nothing there about his current success rate, or personality, however.

Can you learn something about a surgeon from the Classified Telephone Directory? Not much: the specialty, the group if he belongs to a group, sometimes the board certification. Most surgeons haven't taken to advertising yet; though ethically permissible now, it still has an unpleasant odor among the surgical style setters.

You might think it reasonable to ask the surgeon how many operations such as yours he has done and what his results have been. Go ahead, but

---

*ABMS *Compendium of Certified Medical Specialists*, published by the American Board of Medical Specialties, 1986.
Directory of Medical Specialists, Marquis. AMA *Directory*. (Contains only members of the AMA.) American Medical Association.

don't expect to learn the full story. Unless he is planning to publish an article, a surgeon usually doesn't keep up-to-the-minute, follow-up records. Your surgeon may give you the results published in the medical literature and imply that his results will be the same or better. (Actually, when looked into, it turns out that the published mortality rates he quotes are always lower and success rates higher than those actually achieved with an operation.) If a surgeon has done well recently, of course, he will tell you about this, but if he has been having trouble, he'll clam up because he is confident that things are going to look up. Let's hope that things *are* going to look up, but don't bet big money on it.

21

Don't Despair

So that to believe in medicine would be the height of folly, if not to believe in it were not greater folly still, for from this mass of errors there have emerged in the course of time many truths.

MARCEL PROUST,
Guermantes Way

After my previous cautionary chapters, ascribing folly, placing blame, let me turn to the many truths. The medical enterprise is stronger than ever, surgery is safer, and you, the consumer, are better off than you once might have been. Too much surgery still; that has been a central theme of this book, but except in emergencies, the choice for surgery is clearly your choice; you don't have to accept it. Your judgment—sharpened, I hope, by reading this book—will guide you. You can agree to surgery rationally, not as an obedient child, not as a cult parishioner, no longer the lamb.

Let me credit the medical establishment with its good intentions. Most of its members, throughout their range of interests from basic science to clinical practice, sincerely want to help you. You may suffocate in the embrace of their misguided benevolence, but goodwill must be respected tentatively. It's a proper motive for sound medical design.

Although they may never achieve for us our fantasy of perpetual life, the healing professions have lengthened and eased our lives. With the best of their record displayed before us, we expect them to do even better, and they probably will. We admire, envy, revere their work—though excessively, it seems to me. As they provide benefits, they also pander to our enormous health-care appetite. I sometimes wonder if, with totally free choice, the future will not see every citizen as a specialized healer, the entire lot of them mincing back and forth between each other's clinics, taking care of one another.

Scientific medicine *is* better than ever. It has eased surgery's pain and lessened its danger. Diagnosis, made precise by marvelous new instruments, costs more, but it prevents blundering surgical invasions. We now rarely hear of nonemergency exploratory laparotomies. With his CAT scan, NMR, ultrasound, fine needles, and angiograms, the diagnostician plots an accurate map for the surgical campaign. The surgeon no longer attacks a deep cancer with inadequate reconnaissance. To the impatient surgeon, and to the apprehensive patient, diagnostic technology may at times seem no more than cause for money-making delay or as an example of too much "defensive medicine," but it has made surgery more accurate, less frequently useless.

By learning how the body fluids shift, how the composition of blood changes, how the circulation responds, what metabolic alterations occur, and other details of our body's response to injury (or to surgery—a type of injury), surgeons can provide remedies that lower surgical risk. Intravenous fluid administration responds to minute-to-minute need; complex machinery aids breathing and monitors every heartbeat.

The postsurgical intensive care unit with its respirators, heart monitors, computers, special nurses, and special technicians has evolved from sound, basic physiological knowledge. In cases where intensive care has prolonged life hopelessly, it has been criticized justifiably, but its use has made previously untenable surgery now an everyday experience. Operations once high-risk, hair-raising adventures have become routine.

Teams of ingenious medical scientists, allied scientists, engineers, and surgeons have erected surgery's impressive technological edifice. In its rooms surgeons replace hearts, lungs, kidneys; they unplug major vessels, rebuild deformed heads, separate Siamese twins, and straighten noses (without a detectable scar). When needed, surgery is better than ever. If you have chosen it wisely, rejoice.

Anesthesia, under the direction of devoted professionals, contributes mightily to the safety and success of modern surgery. A few years ago a mortality due to general anesthesia of 1 per 1,000 was accepted; now it is 1 per 10,000 or less (Dripps, 1988). Any specific surgical operation is safer than it was a decade ago, and recovery is faster.

Modern surgery's technological enterprise deserves the credit it frequently receives in the news and from its satisfied clients. Its critics refer to improper and excessive use, not to its technological success.

CONTROLLED TESTING—OUTCOME RESEARCH

Though sometimes grudgingly, surgeons are beginning to accept controlled clinical testing of their work. The large breast-surgery studies (Chapter 9) were conceived and directed by surgeons. Smaller controlled clinical tests have been reported frequently. Although it's unlikely that surgical operations can ever be tested as thoroughly as pills are now tested before FDA (Food and Drug Administration) acceptance, controlled testing is on the rise. The insurer, the taxpayer, the critic, and you, the client, will be heard. Gone are the helter-skelter days. In order to attract attention, an enthusiastic surgeon pushing a new idea or a new operation has to come up with sound evidence these days, ideally a random, controlled test. Without it, though his work is published, the surgeon may receive only diffident attention.

With objectives similar to those of controlled clinical testing, patient-outcome research is shedding light on the effectiveness of surgical operations and other medical technologies. Because this research depends on analysis of medical records already available in government, hospital, and insurance-company data banks, rather than on the advanced planning and years of follow-up that clinical testing requires, it is quicker and less expensive. A suitable way of monitoring operations already in widespread use, it has revealed surprising variations and unexpected results in prostate surgery (see Chapter 6). Health-policy specialists hope that it will point the way to containing costs, but it should also help you, the consumer, by providing much better information on doctors and hospitals (Winslow, 1989).

SECOND OPINION

Surgeons learned quickly to live with the second-opinion movement. Why not? They operate in the open for all to see and to second-guess. In contrast to the surgeon's exposure, witness the behavior of other practitioners: Who really knows what goes on in a psychiatrist's consultation room, or what jumble of pills the internist, working alone in his small office, prescribes to what strange effect?

Along with second opinions comes frank disclosure and informed consent. Surgeons tell me that they don't mind this. Takes more talking, but the talking may help clear their own heads, and by bringing the patient more fully into the decision process, they may relieve a little of their own responsibility and gain more patient cooperation. The price is worth paying, and—let's face it—the talk can no longer be avoided.

It's a radically changed world for the doctor: informed consent, second opinion, medical review procedures, strange money sources, a blizzard of paper. Changes as radical, some say, as those that reformed medical education, and thereby the nature of a doctor, seventy-five years ago. Some consequences of any change are unwanted, but in the matter of your interest in avoiding an operation you don't need, or in obtaining one you do need, I think your chances have improved.

DOCTOR SURPLUS

The doctor surplus, certain to continue, even increase, at least for the next decade (Goldsmith, 1986), may or may not help you. Doctor visits should be easier, but not all observers are convinced that more doctor visits are a good thing. David Rogers, of the Robert Wood Johnson Foundation (1977), said that "We need much more solid evidence that a physician visit yields better medical care . . ." Furthermore, unless there is a huge increase in surgery, the presence of more surgeons will mean less-experienced surgeons and more competition. The cooperation characteristic of the best medical practice may suffer, with physicians failing to help one another as readily as they once did.

On the other hand, the surplus may help you by providing more choice, more qualified specialists from whom to choose. Already, board-certified surgeons are found in community hospitals, and soon, you will find just around the corner an expert ready to operate in one of the new surgical outpatient clinics—perhaps (though not soon) at bargain rates.

Personal attention should increase. The most popular doctors may still be able to get away with the long office waits and the brief chats that too frequently define present-day medical etiquette, but in order to stay in business, doctors in oversupply will have to please their customers at all levels of care. Cures will be expected, but the cures, and the failures, may come about as part of a more dignified, courteous, leisurely interaction. Even the poor may discover a finer texture in the doctor-patient exchange. Your doctor may have to learn to behave not only as a scientist and a priest, but as a salesman too.

Will a mass of new MDs, by their numbers and reduced prices, push chiropractors, acupuncturists, and holistic gurus out of store-front offices, and totally dominate the medical scene? Not a likely prospect, perhaps not a desirable one. Until clinical medicine more nearly reaches scientific competence, and its clients abandon their natural human craving for mystical and miraculous cures, wide gaps in the fabric of traditional care will remain open for fringe practitioners, for the medical boonies. Outliers will practice their cults, and MDs, knowingly or unknowingly, will tend, at times, to wave similar incantatory wands.

CHANGES IN PRACTICE

New styles of medical practice may help you, though no one as yet fully understands them or has adequately measured their impact. They may, as in the case of Health Maintenance Organizations (HMOs), slow the surgical momentum, however. HMO providers receive the same yearly fee whether or not they perform surgery, and thus are less likely to recommend surgery.

Medical insurers (private or governmental) and large employers now take a hand in trying to help you—the same hand, albeit, with which they try to conserve their funds. They support patient-outcome research, hire managed-care companies to audit doctors, and require second opinions, because they find that this policy reduces the number of surgeries—presumably eliminating some that are useless.

BAD OPERATIONS IMPROVE—A LITTLE

Just as we have had bad wars, bad economic schemes, bad taxes, and bad politicians, we have had bad operations. They will doubtless remain, but I believe that today's bad operations are not quite as bad as yesterday's. A difficult opinion to defend, I'll admit, for the background of wisdom requires time, and the evidence on today's operations is not in yet. We won't finally make up our minds about them until that time when we will probably look back, shake our heads, sigh, and wonder how so many of them could have been done by rational operators on rational victims.

Nonetheless, do we have anything as silly as goat-gland implants for male impotence? Of course not. A million T&As a year? None of that excess these days. We're becoming sensible. You're still worried about all those hysterectomies, those innumerable cesarean sections, the unnecessary coronary bypasses? So am I. But I find consolation in knowing that these operations are not as dangerous as yesterday's operations were. We have antibiotics now and the technology of life-support. Though you may not *need* a particular operation, your chances of surviving that particular operation are good.

CITIZENS' GROUPS—MEDICAL INDEPENDENCE

As the imperious protector of vital matters, traditional medicine expects sharp criticism. Everyone, from folk-medicine grannies to prize-winning scientists, takes a crack at the medical establishment. Clerks in vitamin emporiums credit themselves with more nutritional wisdom than your doctor. The news media faults emergency rooms, prenatal care, physician greed, the excesses of liposuction, and the shortage of nurses. Philosophers comment on the inflated value doctors attach to an individual life. Politicians raise their eyebrows when asked to spend still more money on the persistently elusive cure for cancer. Why does it take so long to conquer AIDS? And on top of it all, the medical enterprise is so greedy. Can it be that this voracious industry will someday demand more money than our nuclear-bomb business?

Attentive citizens rise up, organize, show interest in all sections and in all fragments of the medical trade and its tools. By joining the right group you can find a midwife, keep up-to-date on nutrition, study ways for living longer, or learn how to die. Citizens' groups, individual writers, and various cultists publish a bulky literature spanning a wide range of medical sense and nonsense. The best is useful, the worst annoying, possibly dangerous.

Most of that vast literature will never be seriously criticized—certainly not by me. If you read it, the reading will call up your own critical sense. As something to consider, however, here is a list of a few of the better lay medical periodicals I see: *Berkeley Wellness Letter, Johns Hopkins Medical Letter, Health After 50, Nutrition Action Healthletter, Prevention, The Edell Health Letter, Mayo Clinic Health Letter, Longevity, Natural Healing Newsletter, Hippocrates, FDA Consumer Health Letter, Tufts University Diet and Nutrition Letter, Omni Longevity, Birthing News*. I find it encouraging that there is enough interest and enthusiasm abroad to spawn so much, often lucid, medical writing.

These publications, which intend to keep you informed, newspapers, popular magazines, and television, indirectly sharpen the medical profession. If a doctor knows that his patients are going to read and ask questions, he must keep informed. The interest of consumer groups, and the focus of the news media (despite its frequent distortions) tend to challenge the physician, force him to provide convincing reasons for his actions, stimulate his continuing education.

If, despite the warnings, examples, and pleas that fill the pages of this book, you still want to try something a little "crazy" in the way of surgery, you may. Though you may have to pay for the choice, we have a free-choice system. You could, for example, still find "psychic surgeons" in the Philippines. (Since psychic surgery doesn't even penetrate the skin, it's not apt to harm you much, except by delay of more effective treatment, should there be any.)

AVOID THE WHOLE MESS, IF POSSIBLE

For most of your life you can avoid the whole complicated, medical mess. A time may come, doubtless will come (perhaps as a surprise), when you need surgical help. Maybe the time is now. But be sure, be cautious.

Personal hygiene, sound nutrition, and exercise, aided by the highest medical technology—vaccines, antibiotics, and public-health measures, are good examples—will usually see our bodies through to their normal life expectancy. Few doctor visits are required. Checkups are for the neurotic, the lonely, and the bored who are then found nibbling pills like popcorn and cowering in the bizarre haven of the surgical suite. Observe, if you will, the prematurely broken and anxious as they spend their days in postoperative physiotherapy, devouring special diets to counteract the damage done by their pills; but don't waste your precious time on all that. Head out, away from the aroma of spilled urine and the rustle of starched white cloth. The somber, earnest face, its mouth spouting the jargon of the helping professions, can propose trouble: Ultrasound may lead to cholecystectomy, an angiogram to a bypass.

Learn to accept. Even the most expensive machinery, the most potent pills, and the most imaginative surgical reconstructions, fail at last in the fight against age. We are not, like automobiles, held together by regular maintenance. Our sparkplugs are irreplaceable.

Surgery can rebuild many imperfections, correct development blunders, open some plugged channels, bypass others, close wounds, remove tumors, fix broken bones, promote natural recovery. It can perform marvels. But don't ask too much of it.

George Crile, Jr., said, "Remember this about surgery: There are risks. There are benefits. There are choices. There are alternatives. It is your body. It is your life. The final decision is yours."

References

ABC TV program. December 16, 1988.

Annexton, M., 1978. "Burrowing through blocked arteries with a balloon 'relocates' plaques." *Journal of the American Medical Association* (henceforth *JAMA*), 240:1117–49.

Applegate, W.B., et al., 1987. "Impact of cataract surgery with lens implantation on vision and physical function in elderly patients." *JAMA*, 275:1064–66.

Asher, R., 1951. "Munchausen's syndrome." *Lancet*, February 10, 339–41.

Aspirin Myocardial Infarction Study Research Group, 1980. "A randomized, controlled trial of aspirin in persons recovered from myocardial infarction." *JAMA*, 243:661–69.

Bailar, J. C. III, and E. M. Smith, 1986. "Progress against cancer?" *New England Journal of Medicine* (henceforth *N Engl J Med*), 314:1226–32.

Bakwin, H. 1958, "The tonsil-adenoidectomy enigma." *Journal of Pediatrics*, 52:339.

Barber, B., 1976. "The ethics of experimentation with human subjects," *Scientific American* (henceforth *Sc Am*), 234 (February): 25–28.

Barnes, D. M., 1987. "Prostate cancer consensus hampered by lack of data," *Science*, 236:1626–27.

Barnett, H. J. M., et al., 1987. "Are the results of extracranial-intracranial bypass trial generalizable?" *N Engl J Med,* 316:820–24.

Barry, M. J., et al., 1988. "Watchful waiting vs. immediate transurethral resection for symptomatic prostatism," *JAMA,* 259:3010–17.

Beardsley, T., 1988. "Radon retried," *Sc Am,* 259:18–19.

Beecher, H. K., 1955. "The powerful placebo," *JAMA,* 159:1602–1606.

———, 1961. "Surgery as placebo," *JAMA,* 176:1102–1107.

———, 1970. *Research and the Individual: Human Studies.* Boston: Little, Brown & Co., 1970.

Benson, H., and D. P. McCallie, Jr., 1979. "Angina pectoris and the placebo effect," *N Engl J Med,* 300:1424–28.

Binder, P. S., 1984. "The status of radial keratotomy in 1984," *Archives of Ophthalmology,* 102:1601–1603.

Block, P.C., 1984. "Mechanism of transluminal angioplasty," *American Journal of Cardiology,* 53:69C–71C.

Boggs, R. J., 1987. "Foreign medical graduates in U.S. surgery," *Bulletin of the American College of Surgeons* (henceforth *Bull Am Coll Surg*), 72:(July) 4–11.

Bolande, R. P., 1969. "Ritualistic surgery—circumcision and tonsillectomy," *N Engl J Med,* 280:591–96.

Bonchek, L. I. 1979. "Are randomized trials appropriate for evaluating new operations?" *N Engl J Med,* 301:44–45.

Booth, W., 1988. "A new way to slice the doctor's pie," *Science,* 242:26.

Bottoms, S. F., et al., 1980. "The increase in the cesarean birth rate," *N Engl J Med,* 302:559–63.

Braunwald, E., 1983, "Effects of coronary-artery bypass grafting on survival," *N Engl J Med,* 309:1181–84.

Bredlau, C. E., et al., 1985. "In-hospital morbidity and mortality in patients undergoing elective coronary angioplasty," *Circulation,* 72:1044–52.

Brody, J. E., 1986. "Children's ear tubes," *Santa Barbara News Press,* October 7.

Brown, J. H., 1986. "Urology: From uromancers to urology." *Bull Am Coll Surg,* 71 (April):17–20.

Bubrick, M. P., and R. B. Benjamin, 1985. "Hemorrhoids and anal fissures," *Postgraduate Medicine* 77 (February):165.

Bullough, P. G., 1983. "Biocompatibility and allogenicity," *Journal of Orthopedic Research* 1:203–205.

Burnett, L. S., 1988a. "Gynecologic history, examination and operations," in H. W. Jones III, et al., eds., *Novak's Textbook of Gynecology*. Baltimore: Williams & Wilkins, 1988, pp. 3–39.

———, 1988b. "Relaxations, malpositions, fistulas, and incontinence," in H. W. Jones III, et al., eds., *Novak's Textbook of Gynecology*. Baltimore: Williams & Wilkins, 1988, pp. 455–78.

Cairns, J., 1985. "The treatment of diseases and the war against cancer," *Sc Am*, 253:51–59.

Califf, R. M., et al., 1989. "The evolution of medical and surgical therapy for coronary artery disease," *JAMA* 261:2077–86.

Campbell, J., 1988. *The Power of Myth*. Garden City, N.Y.: Doubleday, 1988.

Cancer Prevention. Bulletin of U.S. Department of Health and Human Services.

Carden, T. S., Jr., 1978. "Tonsillectomy—trials and tribulations," *JAMA*, 240:1961–62.

Carson, G., 1960. *The Roguish World of Doctor Brinkley*. New York: Rinehart. Co. Inc. 1960.

Carson, R. A., 1977. "What are physicians for?" *JAMA*, 238:1029–31.

CASS principle investigators, 1983. "Coronary artery surgery study (CASS): a randomized trial of coronary artery bypass surgery," *Circulation*, 68:939–50.

Catalona, W. J., and W. W. Scott, 1986. "Carcinoma of the prostate," in P. C. Walsh et al., eds., *Campbell's Urology*, 5th ed. Philadelphia & London: W. B. Saunders, 1986, pp. 1463–1534.

"Cataracts," 1987. *Health Letter*, 3 (March):1–6.

Cheitlin, M.D., 1988. "The aggressive war on acute myocardial infarction: Is the blitzkrieg strategy changing?" *JAMA*, 260:2894–96.

Clarke, J. R., 1985. "A comparison of decision analysis and second opinions for surgical decisions," *Archives of Surgery*, 120:844–47.

Clendening, L., 1942. *Source Book of Medical History*. New York and London: Paul B. Hoeber, 1942.

Condon, R. E., 1986. "Appendicitis," in David C. Sabiston, Jr., ed., *Textbook of Surgery*. Philadelphia: W. B. Saunders, 1986, pp. 967–82.

Conn, D. L., 1983. "Medical considerations regarding indications and contraindications for total hip replacement," *Journal of Orthopedic Research*, 1:190–91.

Consensus Conference, 1987. "The management of clinically localized prostate cancer," *JAMA*, 258:2727–30.

Consensus Conference, 1982. "Total hip-joint replacement in the United States," *JAMA*, 248:1817–24.

Cooke, P., 1987. "Delivery Refused," *Hippocrates*, May/June:63–73.

Corman, M. L., 1988. *Colon and Rectal Surgery*. Philadelphia: J. B. Lippincott Co., 1988.

Council on Scientific Affairs, AMA, 1984. "Early detection of breast cancer," *JAMA*, 252:3008–11.

Cousins, N., 1977. "The mysterious placebo," *Saturday Review*, October 1.

———, 1978. "Medicine as art and philosophy," Address, University of Minnesota, June 2, 1978.

Crile, Grace, ed., 1947. *George Crile*. Philadelphia: Lippincott, 1947.

Crile, G., Jr., 1961. Simplified treatment of cancer of the breast: early results of a clinical study. *Annals of Surgery*, 153:745–61.

———, 1978. *Surgery. Your Choices, Your Alternatives*. New York: Delacorte, 1978.

Crowley, A. E., 1988. "Highlights of the 1988 education issue," *JAMA*, 260:1049–50.

Culliton, B. J., 1987. "GAO report angers cancer officials," *Science*, 236:380–81.

Curran, W. J., 1987. "Medical peer review of physician competence and performance: legal immunity and the antitrust laws," *N Engl J Med*, 316:597–98.

Dateline: Washington, 1987. "Inspector general releases coronary artery bypass graft study," *Bull Am Coll Surg*, 72 (October):2.

Detre, K., et al., 1988. "Percutaneous transluminal coronary angioplasty in 1985–1986 and 1977–1981," *N Engl J Med* 318:265–70.

"Diagnostic and therapeutic technology assessment," (DATTA), 1989. *JAMA*, 261:105–09.

Dicker, R. C., et al., 1982. "Hysterectomy among women of reproductive age," *JAMA*, 248:323–27.

Doll, R., and R. Peto, 1981. *The Causes of Cancer*. Oxford: Oxford University Press, 1981.

Dowling, J. L., and R. L. Bahr, 1985. "A survey of current cataract surgical techniques," *American Journal of Ophthalmology*, 99:35–39.

Dripps, R. D., et al., 1988. *Anesthesia*, 7th ed. Philadelphia: W. B. Saunders, 1988.

Duffey, W. S., Jr., 1988–89. "Radial keratotomy on trial: New surgical procedures and the antitrust laws," *Refractive and Corneal Surgery*, 4:232–40 and 5:27–32.

Durant, J. R. 1987. "Immunotherapy of cancer," *N Engl J Med*, 316:939–40.

Dykes, M. H. M., 1974. "Uncritical thinking in medicine," *JAMA*, 227:1275–77.

Easterday, C. L., et al., 1983. "Hysterectomy in the United States," *Obstetrics and Gynecology*, 62:203–12.

EC/IC Bypass Study Group, 1985. "Failure of extracranial–intracranial arterial bypass to reduce the risk of ischemic stroke," *N Engl J Med*, 313:1191–1200.

Eckberg, T. J., et al., 1987. "Swimming and tympanostomy tubes," *Laryngoscope*, 97:740–41.

ECSS European Coronary Surgery Study Group, 1982. "Prospective randomized study of coronary artery bypass surgery in stable angina pectoris," *Circulation* 65(supplement II):67–71.

Eggleston, J. C., and P. C. Walsh, 1985. "Radical prostatectomy with preservation of sexual function," *Journal of Urology*, 134:1146–48.

Eiseman, B., 1980. *What Are My Chances?* Philadelphia: W. B. Saunders, 1980.

Eisenberg, L., 1977. "The social imperatives of medical research," *Science*, 198:1105–10.

Ejeskar, A., et al., 1983. "Surgery versus chemonucleolysis for herniated lumbar discs," *Clinical Orthopaedics*, No. 174, 236–42.

Ellis, V., 1989. "Public is vulnerable to bad doctors, study says," *L. A. Times*, April 6, I.

Engel, G. L., 1975. "Psychophysiological gastrointestinal disorders," in A. M. Freedman et al., eds., *Comprehensive Textbook of Psychiatry*. Baltimore: Williams & Wilkins, 1975, p. 1643.

Entman, S. S., 1988. "Leiomyoma and adenomyosis," in H. W. Jones III, et al., eds., *Novak's Textbook of Gynecology*. Baltimore: Williams & Wilkins, 1988, pp. 443–54.

Esterday, C. L., et al., 1983. "Hysterectomy in the United States," *Obstetrics and Gynecology*, 62:203–12.

Everson, T., and W. H. Cole, 1966. *Spontaneous Regression of Cancer.* Philadelphia: W. B. Saunders, 1966.

Feldman, A. R., et al., 1986, "The prevalence of cancer," N Engl J Med, 315:1394–97.

Feller, W., et al., 1986. "Modified radical mastectomy with immediate breast reconstruction," *Annals of Surgery*, 52:129.

"Final word on disputed mastectomies," 1978. *Science*, 202:728.

Fink, A. J., 1986. "Letters to editor." N Engl J Med, 315:1167.

Fisher, B., et al., 1985. "Five-year results of a randomized clinical trial comparing total mastectomy and segmental mastectomy, etc.," N Engl J Med 312:665–73.

———, 1985. "Ten-year results of a randomized clinical trial, etc.," N Engl J Med, 312:674–81.

Flye, M. W., 1986, "Disorders of Veins," in David C. Sabiston, Jr., ed., *Textbook of Surgery*. Philadelphia: W. B. Saunders, 1986, p. 1709.

Fogarty, T. J., et al., 1963. "A method for extraction of arterial emboli and thrombi," *Surgery, Gynecology and Obstetrics*, 116:241.

Fowler, F. J., Jr., et al., 1988. "Symptom status and quality of life following prostatectomy," JAMA, 159:3018–22.

Fox, M. S., 1979. "On the diagnosis and treatment of breast cancer," JAMA, 241:489–94.

Freiman, J. A., et al., 1978. "The importance of beta, the type II error and sample size in the design and interpretation of the randomized control trial," N Engl J Med, 299:690–94.

Freidman, E., 1984. "Second-opinion programs come into their own," *Hospitals*, July 16, 105–108.

Fry, J., 1957. "Are all 'T's and A's' really necessary?" *British Medical Journal*, 1:124–29.

Fry, T. L., and H. C. Pillsbury, 1987. "The implications of 'controlled' studies of tonsillectomy and adenoidectomy," *Otolaryngological Clinics of North America*, 20:409–13.

Frymoyer, J. W., 1988. "Back pain and sciatica," N Engl J Med, 318:291–300.

Garrison, F. H., 1929. *An Introduction to the History of Medicine.* Philadelphia: W. B. Saunders, 1929.

Gates, G. A., et. al. 1987, "Effectiveness of adenoidectomy and tympanostomy tubes in the treatment of chronic otitis media with effusion," *N Engl J Med*, 317:1444–51.

Gibbon, R. P., et al., 1984. "Total prostatectomy for localized prostatic cancer," *Journal of Urology*, 131:73–76.

Glassow, M. A., 1987. "The Shouldice repair for inguinal hernia," in L. M. Nyhus and R. E. Condon, eds., *Hernia*. Philadelphia: J. P. Lippincott, 1987, pp. 163–78.

Glen, F., 1983. "Silent or asymptomatic gallstones," in J. P. Delaney and R. L. Varco, eds., *Controversies in Surgery II*. Philadelphia: W. B. Saunders, 1983, pp. 355–61.

Goldsmith, J. C., 1986. "The U.S. health care system in the year 2000," *JAMA*, 256:3371–75.

Goldsmith, M. F., 1985. "*Caveat emptor* tops the eye chart for radial keratotomy candidates," *JAMA*, 254:3401–3403.

———, 1988. "Artery-expanding stents widen hope for patients with atherosclerosis," *JAMA*, 259:327–29.

———, 1989. "New visceral transplants invigorate cancer victims," *JAMA*, 261:1397.

Goldwyn, R. M., 1987. "Current concepts. Breast reconstruction after mastectomy." *N Engl J Med*, 317:1711–14.

Gomez-Marin, O., et al., 1987. "Improvement in long-term survival among patients hospitalized with acute myocardial infarction, 1970 to 1980," *N Engl J Med*, 316:1353–59.

Gordon, R., 1983. *Great Medical Disasters*. New York: Dorset Press, 1983.

Goyert, G. L., et al., 1989. "The physician factor in cesarean birth rates," *N Engl J Med*, 320:706–709.

Graboys, T. B., et al., 1987. "Results of a second-opinion program for coronary artery bypass graft surgery," *JAMA*, 258:1611–14.

Graboys, T. B., 1989. "Conflicts of interest in the management of silent ischemia," *JAMA*, 261:2116–17.

Graham, H., 1939. *The Story of Surgery*. New York: Doubleday, Doran & Co, 1939.

Grayhack, J. T., et al., eds., 1976. *Benign Prostatic Hyperplasia*. Bethesda, Md.: Department of Health, Education and Welfare, 1976.

Greenfield, S., 1989. "The state of outcome research: Are we on target?" *N Engl J Med*, 320:1142–43.

Grossman, E., and N. A. Posner, 1981. "Surgical circumcision of neonates: a history of its development." *Obstetrics and Gynecology*, 58:241–46.

Grotta, J. C., 1987. "Current medical and surgical therapy for cerebrovascular disease," *New Engl J Med*, 317:1505–16.

Grüntzig, A. R., et al, 1979. "Nonoperative dilatation of coronary-artery stenosis," *N Engl J Med*, 301:61–68.

Guerci, A. D., et al., 1987. "A randomized trial of intravenous tissue plasminogen activator for acute myocardial infarction with subsequent randomization to elective coronary angioplasty," *N Engl J Med*, 317:1613–18.

Gunby, P., 1980. "For cancer, the good news is survival; the bad news is incidence," *JAMA*, 243:1789–90.

———, 1983. "Chymopapain: tropical tree to surgical suite," *JAMA*, 249:1115–23.

———, 1987. "Laser may provide better channel, smoother lumen in future coronary arterial occlusions; full potential awaits improved technology," *JAMA*, 257:1283.

Gundle, M. J., et al., 1980. "Psychosocial outcome after coronary artery surgery," *American Journal of Psychiatry*, 137:1591.

Haggerty, R. J., 1968. "Diagnosis and treatment: tonsils and adenoids—a problem revisited," *Pediatrics*, 41:815–17.

Hancock, B. D., and K. Smith, 1975. "The internal sphincter and Lord's procedure for haemorrhoids," *British Journal of Surgery*, 62:833–36.

Haynes de Regt, R., et al., 1986. "Relation of private or clinic care to the cesarean birth rate," *N Engl J Med*, 315:619–24.

"Help for Stroke Victims," 1987. *Longevity*, April, p. 60.

Hiatt, H. H., 1977. "Lessons of the coronary-bypass debate," *N Engl J Med*, 297:1462–64.

Horowitz, L. C., 1988. *Taking Charge of Your Medical Fate*. New York, Random House, 1988.

Huggins, C., et al., 1941. "Studies on prostatic cancer—II, the effects of castration on advanced carcinoma of the prostate gland," *Archives of Surgery*, 43:209.

Jacobi, G. H., and R. Hohenfellner, eds., 1982. *Prostate Cancer*. Baltimore: Williams and Wilkins, 1982.

Javid, M. J., 1983. "Safety and efficacy of chymopapain (chymodiactin) in herniated nucleus pulposus with sciatica," *JAMA*, 249:2489–94.

Jewett, H. J., 1975. "The present status of radical prostatectomy for stages A and B prostatic cancer," *Urological Clinics of North America*, 2:105.

Jonas, H. S., 1987. "The torch is passed: Editorial," *JAMA*, 258:3554–55.

Kelsey, J. L., 1983. "Total hip joint replacement: epidemiology and impact," *Journal of Orthopedic Research*, 1:196–68.

Kent, K. M., 1987. "Coronary angioplasty. A decade of experience," *N Engl J Med*, 316:1148–50.

Keys, A. and M., 1959. *Eat Well and Stay Well*. Garden City: Doubleday, 1959.

Kirn, T. F., 1987a. "Long-term study evidence accumulating, but radial keratotomy controversy continues: Medical News & Perspectives," *JAMA*, 257:1282.

———, 1987b. "Ophthalomology's new tools may have profound impact on refractive surgery, Medical News & Perspectives." *JAMA*, 257:2129–30.

———, 1987c. "Orthopedic surgeons ponder: how best to secure artificial hip prostheses." *JAMA*, 258:173.

———, 1989. "Atheroma curettage: An idea whose time may come as several devices begin trials," *JAMA*, 261:498–89.

Kolata, G., 1981. "Consensus on bypass surgery," *Science*, 211:42–43.

———, 1983. "Some bypass surgery unnecessary." *Science*, 222:605–606.

Krantz, P., 1986. "When your best bet is to get a second opinion," *Better Homes and Gardens*, 64: (February) 70.

Kunz, J., 1977. "Mammography dispute continues to simmer: Medical World News," *JAMA*, 238:1999–2006.

Leveno, K. J., et al., 1986. "A prospective comparison of selective and universal electronic fetal monitoring in 34,995 pregnancies," *N Engl J Med*, 315:615–19.

Lord, P. H., 1968. "A new regime for the treatment of haemorrhoids," *Proceedings of the Royal Society of Medicine*, 61:935–86.

Love, J. W., 1975. "Drugs and operations," *JAMA*, 232:37–38.

Luchi, R. J., et al., 1987. "Comparison of medical and surgical treatment for unstable angina pectoris," *N Engl J Med*, 316:977–84.

Lytton, B., 1988. "Urology. What's new in surgery," *Bull Am Coll Surg*, 73 (February):42–50.

Mackenzie, N. A., 1974. *The Magic of Rudolph Valentino*. London: Research Publishing, 1974.

Mandel, E. M., et al., 1987. "Efficacy of amoxicillin with and without decongestant-antihistamine for otitis media with effusion in children," *N Engl J Med*, 316:432–7.

Manniche, C., et al., 1988. "Clinical trial of intensive muscle training for chronic low back pain," *Lancet*, December 24, pp. 1473–76.

Martini, C. J. M., 1988. "Evaluating the competence of health professionals," *JAMA*, 260:1057–8.

Marx, J. L., 1988. "Which clot-dissolving drug is best?" *Science*, 242:1505–1506.

Maugh, T. II, 1978. "Chemical carcinogens: The scientific basis for regulation," *Science*, 201:1200–5.

Maugh, T. II, 1982, "Cancer is not inevitable," *Science*, 217:36–7.

Mayer, R. J., and W. B. Patterson, 1988. "How is cancer treatment chosen?" *N Engl J Med*, 318:636–8.

McCarthy, E. G., and G. W. Widmer, 1974. "Effects of screening by consultants on recommended elective surgical procedures," *N Engl J Med*, 291:1331–5.

McConnell, J. C., and I. T. Khubchandani, 1983. "Long-term follow-up of closed hemorrhoidectomy," *Diseases of the Colon and Rectum*, 26:797

McDonald, M. B., et al., 1987. "The nationwide study of epikeratophakia for myopia," *American Journal of Ophthalmology*, 103:375–83.

McPherson, D. D., et al., 1987. "Delineation of the extent of coronary atherosclerosis by high-frequency epicardial echocardiography," *N Engl J Med*, 316:304–309.

McWhirter, R., 1948. "The value of simple mastectomy and radiotherapy in the treatment of cancer of the breast," *British Journal of Radiology*, 21:599–610.

Meade, R. H., 1968. *An Introduction to the History of General Surgery*. Philadelphia: W. B. Saunders, 1968.

Medical Journal Bulletins, 1987. "Second opinion on bypass surgery," *Health Letter*, November 12, p. 11.

Medicine and Health, 1987, *Wall St Jour*, April 24.

Mencken, H. L., 1927. "Dives into quackery: Chiropractic," *Prejudices*. Series 6. New York: Alfred A. Knopf, 1927, pp. 217–27.

Merz, B., 1986. "Antitumor strategies based on enhancing—and blocking—effects of interleukin-2," *JAMA*, 256:1241–4.

————, 1987. "General Accounting Office report on cancer survival statistics raises NCI hackles," *JAMA*, 257:2692–3.

Meyers, W. C., 1986. "Neoplasms of the liver," in *Textbook of Surgery*, edited by David C. Sabiston, Jr., 1079–92. Philadelphia: W. B. Saunders, 1986.

Middleton, R. G., et al., 1986. "Patient survival and local recurrence rate following radical prostatectomy for prostatic carcinoma," *Journal of Urology*, 136:422–24.

Minkoff, H. L., and R. H. Schwarz, 1980. "The rising cesarean section rate: Can it safely be reversed?" *Obstetrics and Gynecology*, 56:135–43.

Mock, M. B., 1984. "Summary: Acute and chronic outcome of percutaneous transluminal coronary angioplasty," *American Journal of Cardiology*, 53:67C–68C.

Moxley, J. H., et al., 1980. "Treatment of primary breast cancer," *JAMA*, 244:797–800.

Mueller, B. A., et al., 1986. "Appendectomy and the risk of tubal infertility," *N Engl J Med*, 315:1506.

Murphy, M. L., 1977. "Treatment of chronic stable angina," *N Engl J Med*, 297:621–27.

Myers, S. A., and N. Gleicher, 1988. "A successful program to lower cesarean-section rates," *N Engl J Med*, 319:1511–16.

Nahrwold, D. L., 1986. "The biliary system," in David C. Sabiston, Jr., eds. *Textbook of Surgery*. Philadelphia: W. B. Saunders, 1986, pp. 1128–61.

Newell, F. W., 1982. *Ophthalmology*, 5th ed. St. Louis: C. V. Mosby, 1982.

"NIH consensus development task force statement on cesarean childbirth," 1989. *American Journal of Obstetrics and Gynecology*, 139:902–909.

Norman, C., 1985. "Clinical trial stirs legal battles," *Science*, 227:1316–18.

Notzon, F. C., et al., 1987. "Comparisons of national cesarean-section rates," *N Engl J Med*, 316:386–89.

Nyhus, L. M., and C. T. Bombeck, 1986. "Hernias," in David C. Sabiston, Jr., ed., *Textbook of Surgery*. Philadelphia: W. B. Saunders, 1986, pp. 1231–51.

Nyhus, L. M., and R. E. Condon, eds., 1978. *Hernia*, 2nd ed. Philadelphia: J. B. Lippincott Company, 1978.

Olsen, K. D., 1986. "Myringotomy tubes—another viewpoint," *Pediatrics* 77:439–41.

O'Mailey, M. S., and S. W. Fletcher, 1987. "Screening for breast cancer with breast self-examination," *JAMA*, 257:2197–2203.

Ornish, D. M., et al., 1988. "Can life-style changes reverse atherosclerosis?" *Circulation*, 78 (Supplement II):10.

Parachini, A., 1988. "Pediatricians group may ease its opposition to circumcision," *LA Times*, June 21.

Parachini, A., 1989. "Circumcision: clear benefits, some risks," *LA Times* V, March 6.

Parella, M. M., 1980. "The middle ear effusions," Parella, M. M. and Shumrick, D., eds., *Otolaryngology*, Philadelphia: W. B. Saunders, 1980, pp. 1422–44.

Pariza, M. W., 1984. "A perspective on diet, nutrition, and cancer." *JAMA*, 251:1455–58.

Perrin, T., et al., 1985. "Functional evaluation of total hip arthroplasty with five- to ten-year follow-up evaluation," *Clinical Orthopedics*, 195:252–59.

Perry, M. C., et al., 1987. "Chemotherapy with or without radiation therapy in limited small-cell carcinoma of the lung," *N Eng J Med*, 316:912–18.

Perry, S., 1978. "From the NIH. The biomedical research community: its place in consensus development," *JAMA*, 239:485–8.

Pickleman, J., and A. L. Schueneman, 1987. "The use and abuse of neuropsychological tests to predict operative performance." *Bull Am Coll Surg*, 72:(February) 7–11.

Plotnick, G. D., 1978. "Medical management of the patient with unstable angina," *JAMA*, 239:860–62.

Preston, F. W., and A. F. Fritz, 1983. "The vermiform appendix," in Harry S. Goldsmith's *Practice of Surgery*. Philadelphia: Harper & Row, 1983. Vol. 2, Chapter 8.

Prevention Guide to Surgery and Its Alternatives. Emmaus, Pa.:Rodale Press, 1980.

Prichard, J. A., et al., 1985. *Williams Obstetrics*. Norwalk, Conn.:Appleton-Century-Crofts, 1985.

"Prostate," 1987. *Health Letters*, 3 (April)1–5.

Puylaert, J. B. C. M., et al., 1987. "A prospective study of ultrasonography in the diagnosis of appendicitis," *N Engl J Med*, 317:666–69.

Rapaport, E., 1989. "Thrombolytic agents in acute myocardial infarction," *N Eng J Med*, 320:861–863.

Relman, A. S., 1987. "The extracranial-intracranial arterial bypass study," *N Engl J Med*, 316:809–10.

———, 1989. "Adjuvant treatment of early breast cancer," *N Engl J Med*, 320:525.

Resnick, M. I., 1989. "Urology," *Bull Am Coll Surg*, 74(February): 40–56.

Robinson, J. C., et al., 1987. "Market and regulatory influences on the availability of coronary angioplasty and bypass surgery in U.S. hospitals," *N Engl J Med*, 317:85–90.

Rooks, J., and J. E. Hass, 1986. *Nurse-midwifery in America*, Washington: American College of Nurse-Midwives Foundation, 1986.

Roos, N. P., et al., 1989, "Mortality and reoperation after open and transurethral resection of the prostate for benign prostatic hyperplasia," *N Engl J Med*, 320:1120–24.

Rosenberg, S. A., et al., 1987. "A progress report on the treatment of 157 patients with advanced cancer using lymphokine-activated killer cells and interleukin-2 or high-dose interleukin-2 alone." *N Engl J Med*, 316:889–97.

Roth, P., 1986. *The Counterlife*. New York: Farrar, Straus, Giroux, 1986.

Rozanski, A., et al., 1988. "Mental stress and the induction of silent myocardial ischemia in patients with coronary artery disease," *N Engl J Med*, 318:1005–12.

Rutkow, I. M., 1986. "General surgical operations in the United States," *Archives of Surgery*, 121:1145–49.

Sackett, D. L., 1980. "The competing objectives of randomized trials," *N Engl J Med*, 303:1059–60.

Sackmann, M., et al., 1988. "Shock-wave lithotripsy of gallbladder stones," *N Engl J Med*, 318:393–97.

Sampson, P., 1978. "Chymopapain: A case study in federal drug regulation," *JAMA*, 240:195–219.

Sandberg, S. I., et al., 1985. "Elective hysterectomy. Benefits, risks, and costs." *Medical Care*, 23:1067–85.

Sattilaro, A. J., 1982. *Recalled by Life*. Boston: Houghton Mifflin, 1982.

Schafer, A., 1982. "The ethics of the randomized clinical trail," *N Engl J Med*, 307:719–24.

Schlossberg, S. M., et al., 1984. "Second opinion for urologic surgery," *Journal of Urology*, 131:209–12.

Schnitt, S. J., et al., 1988. "Current concepts. Ductal carcinomas in situ (intraductal carcinoma) of the breast," N Engl J Med, 318:898–903.

Schoen, E. J., 1987. "Letter to the editor." American Journal of Diseases of Children, 141:128.

Shader, D., 1987. "Soviets pioneer new eye treatment," LA Times, November 27, 1987, V-4.

Shannon, N., and A. Paul, 1979. "L4/5 and L5/S1 disc protrusions: analysis of 323 cases operated on over 12 years," Journal of Neurology, Neurosurgery, and Psychiatry, 42:804–809.

Shiono, P. H., et al., 1987. "Recent trends in cesarean birth and trial of labor rates in the United States," JAMA, 257:494–97.

Showstack, J. A., et al., 1987. "Association of volume with outcome of coronary artery bypass graft surgery," JAMA, 257:785–89.

Sider, R. C., and C. D. Clements, 1985. "The new medical ethics," Archives of Internal Medicine, 145:2169–71.

Siegel, B. S., 1986. Love, Medicine & Miracles. Harper & Row, 1986.

Sigwart, U., et al., 1987. "Intravascular stents to prevent occlusion and restenosis after transluminal angioplasty," N Engl J Med, 316:701–706.

Simmons, J. C. H., 1980. "Lesions of lumbar intervertebral discs," in A. H. Crenshaw, ed., Campbell's Operative Orthopaedics, 6th ed. St. Louis: C. V. Mosby, 1980, p. 2107.

Simonton, O. C., 1978. Getting Well Again. Los Angeles: J. P. Tarcher, Inc., 1978.

Smart, C. R., 1982. "Preventing cancer in the United States," Bull Am Coll Surg, September, 2–8.

Speert, H., 1986. "Historical highlights." in D. N. Danforth and J. R. Scott, eds., Obstetrics and Gynecology. Philadelphia: J. B. Lippincott, 1986.

Spodick, D. H., 1975. "Numerators without denominators. There is no FDA for the surgeon," JAMA, 232:35–36.

Stang, H. J., et al., 1988. "Local anesthesia for neonatal circumcision," JAMA, 259:1507–11.

Stickler, G. B., 1984. "The attack on the tympanic membrane," Pediatrics, 74:291–92.

Stoline, A., and J. P. Weiner, 1988. The New Medical Marketplace. Baltimore: The Johns Hopkins Univ. Press.

Sturdevant, R. A. L, 1977. "How should results of controlled trials affect clinical practice?" Gastroenterology 73:1179–81.

Subcommittee on Oversight and Investigations, 1978. *Surgical Performance: Necessity and Quality*. Washington, D.C.: U.S. Government Printing Office, 1978.

Surgery in the United States, 1975. Am Coll Surg and Am Surg Asc.

Thistle, J. L., et al., 1989. "Dissolution of cholesterol gallbladder stones by methyl *tert*-butyl ether administered by percutaneous transhepatic catheter," N Engl J Med, 320:633–39.

Thomas, D. P., 1969. "Experiment versus authority," N Engl J Med, 281:932–34.

Thomas, L., 1971. "The technology of medicine," N Engl J Med, 285:1366–68.

Thompson, J. P. S., 1977. "Hemorrhoidectomy. How I do it," *Diseases of the Colon and Rectum*, 20:173.

Thomson, W. H. F., 1975. "The nature of haemorrhoids," *British Journal of Surgery*, 62:542–52.

TIMI Research Group, 1988. "Immediate vs. delayed catheterization and angioplasty following thrombolytic therapy for acute myocardial infarction," JAMA, 260:2849–58.

———, 1989. "Comparison of invasive and conservative strategies after treatment with intravenous tissue plasminogen activator in acute myocardial infarction," N Engl J Med, 320:618–27.

Topol, E. J., et al., 1987. "A randomized trial of immediate versus delayed elective angioplasty after intravenous tissue plasminogen activator in acute myocardial infarction," N Engl J Med, 317:581–18.

U.S. Dept. of Health and Human Services, 1986. *Detailed Diagnoses and Procedures for Patients Discharged from Short-stay Hospitals*. Series 13, No. 95. Washington: U.S. Government Printing Office, 1986.

Veterans Administration Co-op, Urological Research Group, 1967. "Treatment and survival of patients with cancer of the prostate," *Surgery, Gynecology and Obstetrics*. 124:1011–17.

Walsh, P. C., 1986. "Benign prostatic hypertrophy," in P. C. Walsh et al., eds., *Campbell's Urology*, 5th ed. Philadelphia & London: W. B. Saunders, 1986, pp. 1248–1265.

Walter, H. J., et al., 1988. "Modification of risk factors for coronary heart disease," N Engl J Med, 318:1093–100.

Wangensteen, O. H., and S. D., 1978. *The Rise of Surgery*. Minneapolis: Universary of Minnesota Press, 1978.

Weber, H., 1983. "Lumbar disc herniation," *Spine*, 8:131–40.

Weinberg, R. A., 1983. "A molecular basis of cancer," *Sc Am*, November, 126–42.

Weinerth, J. L, 1986. "The male genital system," in David C. Sabiston, Jr., ed., *Textbook of Surgery*, Philadelphia: W. B. Saunders, 1986, pp. 1670–95.

Welch, C. E., and R. A. Malt, 1987. "Surgery of the stomach duodenum, gallbladder, and bile ducts," *N Engl J Med*, 316:999–1008.

Wennberg, J. E., et al., 1988. "An assessment of prostatectomy for benign urinary tract obstruction," *JAMA* 259:3027–30.

Wentz, A. C., 1988. "Endometriosis," in H. W. Jones III et al., eds., *Novak's Textbook of Gynecology*. Baltimore: Williams & Wilkins, 1988, pp. 303–27.

Wexler, L., et al., 1989. "The vascular war of 1988," *JAMA* 261:418–19.

White, H. D., et al., 1989. "Effect of intravenous streptokinase as compared with that of tissue plasminogen activator on left ventricular function after first myocardial infarction," *N Engl J Med*, 320:817–21.

Willett, W. C., and B. MacMahon, 1984. "Diet and cancer—an overview," *N Engl J Med*, 310:633–38, 697–703.

Williams, G. R., 1983. "A history of appendicitis," *Annals of Surgery*, 197:495–506.

Willman, V. L., 1984. "Summary: Future research directions," *American Journal of Cardiology*, 53:146C.

Wilson, R. E., 1986. "The Breast," in David C. Sabiston, Jr., ed., *Textbook of Surgery*. Philadelphia: W. B. Saunders, 1986, pp. 530–72.

Winslow, C. M., et al. 1988a, "The appropriateness of performing coronary artery bypass surgery," *JAMA*, 260:505–509.

———, 1988b. "The appropriateness of carotid endarterectomy," *N Engl J Med*, 318:721–27.

Winslow, R., 1989. "Patient data may reshape health care," *Wall Street Journal*, April 17, B1.

Wiswell, T. E., and J. D. Roscelli, 1986. "Corraborative evidence for the decreased incidence of urinary tract infections in circumcised male infants," *Pediatrics*, 78:96–99.

Wolf, S., 1959. "Pharmacology of placebos," *Pharmacology Review*, 11:689–704.

Workshop on Tonsillectomy and Adenoidectomy, 1975. *Annals of Otology Rhinology, and Laryngology*, 84 (supplement 19).

Wright, M. R., 1986. "Surgical addiction," *Archives Otolaryngology and Head and Neck Surgery*, 112:870–72.

Zarins, C. K., 1989. "The vascular war of 1988: The enemy is met," *JAMA*, 261:416–17.

Zimmer, P. J, 1977. "Modern ritualistic surgery," *Clinical Pediatrics*, 16:503–506.

Zimmerman, L. M., and Veith, I., 1961. *"Great Ideas in the History of Surgery."* Baltimore: Williams & Wilkins, 1961.

Index

APSAC (anisoylated plasminogen streptokinase actovator complex), 27
Abdominal cancer, 15
Abscesses, 122, 130
Acupuncture, 147–48, 198–99
Acute cholecystitis, 109–10, 111
Adenoidectomy, 194, 195, 196
    see also Tonsillectomy and Adenoidectomy
Adenoids, 187, 192
Adhesions, 84, 88, 90, 117
Adjuvant treatment (cancer), 101, 176–78
Adrenal gland, 16, 69
Adrenalectomy, 68–69, 104–5
Age, 42
    and prostrate trouble, 57, 58, 59, 65
Aging, 3, 7, 247
    and cataracts, 161
    and impotence, 62
    and surgical competence, 234
    and total hip replacement,
    and varicose veins, 46
Alcohol, 171, 183
American Academy of Orthopaedic Surgeons, 146
American Academy of Pediatrics, 190–91, 192

American Association of Neurological Surgeons, 146
American Board of Surgery, 230
American Cancer Society, 172, 181
American College of Obstetricians and Gynecologists, 90, 190
American College of Surgeons, 66, 231
American Heart Association, 25, 114
American Medical Association (AMA), 231
American Neurological Association, 42–43
American Surgical Association, 231
American Urological Association, Circumcision Study Group, 191
Anal dilatation, 54–55
Anal fistula, 51–52
Anaphylactic shock, 146
Anesthesia, 11, 73, 95, 109, 127, 168, 242–43
Angina, 22, 24, 26, 204, 205
    surgical relief of, 35, 36
Angiography, 39, 242
Angioplasty, 32–33, 37, 209
Animal Rights Movement, 199
Antibiotics, 3, 9, 12, 15, 73, 117
    prophylactic, 121, 122, 123, 153
    in treatment of ear infection, 193, 194
Appendectomy, 13, 115–23
    alternatives to, 122–23